Christine Hill is a physiotherapist. After originally qualifying at St Mary's Hospital, London, as a general physiotherapist she pursued postgraduate training firstly in paediatric and then in obstetric physiotherapy. This makes her one of less than a handful of physiotherapists with both specialist qualifications. She worked at Paddington Green Children's Hospital for ten years, during which time she was trained in both normal and abnormal child development by the Bobaths themselves at the London Bobath Centre. Eventually she became co-superintendent of the children's physiotherapy department at Paddington Green. She subsequently trained as an obstetric physiotherapist and qualified as a full member of the Association of Chartered Physiotherapists in Obstetrics and Gynaecology in 1981. She has run private antenatal and postnatal classes in London for the last sixteen years and sees about 100 women and their babies a week.

Peter Hill is a professor of psychiatry and a consultant child and adolescent psychiatrist at St George's Hospital, London. He is Chairman of the Specialist Section of Child and Adolescent Psychiatry of the Royal College of Psychiatrists. After training as a doctor at Cambridge University and St Bartholomew's Hospital, London, he subsequently worked in various areas of medicine including gastroenterology, paediatric surgery and neurology. He then trained as a psychiatrist at the Maudsley Hospital, eventually specialising in children's psychiatry. He teaches medical students, general practitioners and hospital doctors about child development and children's psychological disorders. One of his research interests is the importance of early treatment interventions with families who have very young children. He has written, edited or co-authored five books on child psychiatry and developmental paediatrics as well as being the author of numerous scientific papers and chapters on children's medicine and child development. He likes parents and hates superficial theorising about children's development.

Christine and Peter Hill are married to each other and have three children.

YOUR NEW BABY
How to survive the first months of parenthood

Christine and Peter Hill

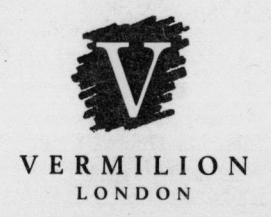

VERMILION
LONDON

First published in the United Kingdom
by Vermilion in 1996

Copyright © 1995 Christine & Peter Hill

The moral right of the authors has been asserted

All rights reserved

No part of this publication may be reproduced, stored in a retrieval system, or transmitted, in any form or by any means without the prior permission in writing of the publisher, nor be otherwise circulated in any form of binding or cover other than that in which it is published and without a similar condition including this condition being imposed on the subsequent purchaser

A CIP catalogue for this book is available from the British Library

ISBN 0 09 181307 7

Typeset by Solidus (Bristol) Limited
Printed and bound in Great Britain by
Mackays of Chatham, Chatham, Kent

Vermilion
An imprint of Ebury Press
Random House UK Ltd
20 Vauxhall Bridge Road
London SW1V 2SA

Contents

Acknowledgements ... xi
First remarks ... 1

STAGE 1 THINKING AHEAD

Thinking ahead ... 7
It's not going to change my life! (Or is it?) ... 9
Work and when to stop it ... 17
   Holidays ... 21
   Thinking ahead about money ... 21
Antenatal classes ... 23
Exercise during pregnancy ... 29
   Pelvic floor muscles ... 30
   How to do it ... 32
   Your back and your front ... 34
Thinking ahead about yourself as a new mother ... 45
   Organising support ... 45
   Organising events around the birth period ... 48
Thinking ahead about your baby ... 51
   The layette (baby gear and equipment) ... 52
   Where is the baby going to sleep? ... 53
   Decisions about feeding ... 54
   Names ... 56
   Circumcision ... 57
Thinking ahead about your other (step-)children ... 59

STAGE 2 IN HOSPITAL

The first hour or so	63
The 'bonding' business	69
Getting it right and the myth of the perfect start	73
The postnatal ward	77
Your pelvic floor	78
How best to help your recovery	79
Lochia	80
Picking up your baby	81
Visitors	82
Starting to breast feed your baby	84
Engorgement	86
Continuing to try to breast feed your baby	87
One breast or two?	87
How often?	88
How long?	88
Sitting in a comfortable position to feed	89
Afterpains	91
Bottle feeding	91
Your first bath	91
Postnatal exercises	92
Baby blues/maternity blues/three-day blues	93
Some other people	94

STAGE 3 AT HOME

Coming home: the first few days	97
(Step-)brothers and sisters	100
Rest	100
Visitors	102
Where will the baby go?	103
In what position should the baby sleep?	106
Your baby	107
Feeding generally	108
Breast feeding	109

Supply and demand 109
Technique 110
Timing 111
Common breast-feeding problems 112
  Sore nipples 112
  Not enough milk? 114
  Your baby doesn't suck 114
Bottle feeding 115
Dummies 116

STAGE 4 LIFE IN THE SLOW AND MIDDLE LANES

One to three weeks: life in the slow lane 121
  Exercises 124
  Feeding (and vomiting) 126
  Changing nappies 128
  Washing and bathing 130
Three to six weeks: life in the middle lane 133
  Your baby's personality 136
  Coping with a crying baby 141
  Evening fretting 145
  Crying which will not stop 149
  Feeding 153
  Mastitis 155

STAGE 5 NUDGING BACK INTO THE FAST LANE

Six weeks onwards: nudging back into the fast lane 161
  Six-week check 161
  Sex 162
  Maintaining your relationship with your husband 163
  Maintaining your social network 166
  Fatigue 167
  Depression 169
  Good habits 172
  Feeding 172

Daytime sleeps 174
Helping your baby to sleep through the night(!) 175
Talking to your baby 177
Developmental checks 179
Immunisation 180
Your weight 181
The elevator exercise 183
Thinking ahead about returning to work 184

STAGE 6 BACK IN THE FAST LANE AND PICKING UP SPEED

Three months onwards 191
  Going back to work 193
    When to return 193
    Childcare arrangements 194
    Full-time or part-time work? 196
  Maintaining your relationship with your husband 196
  Maintaining yourself 199
    Getting some rest 199
    Getting organised 199
    Maintaining your networks 199
  Medical checks 200
  Weaning on to solid food 200
  Dummies 202
  Sleeping 202
  Parenting 204
  Coda 207

SECTION 7 APPENDICES

1. Maternity nurses and nannies 211
2. Layette (small baby gear) 215
3. Big baby equipment 217
4. What to pack for hospital 223
5. Circumcision 225

6. Postnatal exercises	227
7. The perfect pelvic floor	229
8. Is my baby ill?	231
9. Accidents and Basic Principles of First Aid	233
10. Further reading	235
11. Useful addresses	237
Index	239

Acknowledgements

Most of this book was written at Michael and Marty Wolff's remote house in Wiltshire and we are extremely grateful to them for their generosity. On two occasions we were able to borrow Sally and Nick Turquet's house in Cornwall and we would like to thank them too.

A number of people provided critical comments of a remarkably incisive yet courteous quality. We would particularly like to thank: Dr Jake Mackinnon, Consultant Paediatrician, The Portland Hospital for Women and Children; Professor David Hall, Professor of Community Paediatrics, University of Sheffield; Mr Ian Fergusson, Consultant Obstetrician, St Thomas's Hospital; and Mrs Barbara Whiteford, Obstetric and Paediatric Physiotherapist.

In addition we would also like to thank others who took the time to read and make detailed comments on manuscript drafts: Mrs Clare Byam-Cook, Midwife and Feeding Counsellor; Dr Amanda Northridge and Dr Tim Evans, General Practitioners; Dr Robin Basu, Dr Anne Cremona, Dr Tony Jaffa and Dr Alan McClelland – Psychiatrists; Mrs Emma Robarts, Mrs Julie Aldridge, Mrs Clare Seed, Ms Melanie Hall, Mrs Katrina Williams and Mrs Deirdre Skip.

Penny Maddon was kind enough to take several photographs. Araminta Whitley's help was valuable as the manuscript neared completion.

We have appreciated everyone's comments and responded to nearly all of them but the responsibility for the book's contents is finally ours.

First remarks

This is a book for people who know they are not going to need it.

It is for first-time mothers: particularly women who are used to running their own lives and have successful jobs, careers or lifestyles.

Its focus is the first few months after a baby's birth but it is not so much about the babies themselves as about the adults who look after them, about becoming a parent. It is written mainly for mothers and is usually addressed to them, though some sections are for fathers.

We have written it with this focus because we think that although there are some very good baby books, there is no adequate book which might help with the process of becoming a parent when you have not been one before. The first few weeks after birth is a time when most people are very likely to feel rather helpless and useless in their role as new parents: something they had never expected. For people who are normally highly competent and successful, feelings of helplessness may be an unfamiliar experience and therefore a doubly unpleasant one.

Much has been written about how to look after babies but precious little about how new parents can look after themselves. We think they have been overlooked. A pregnant woman is the centre of attention until her baby is born, at which point it is the baby who becomes the focus of everyone's interest. He becomes centre stage and she is displaced to the wings.

The transition to motherhood is made infinitely easier by thinking ahead in a constructive manner. There are, therefore, a few sections which are best read when you are pregnant to enable you to plan.

We have tried to keep it easy to read because we notice, and remember, that pregnancy and the first weeks of parenthood are not the time for digesting complicated texts.

Nobody has found a way round the problem of how to talk about gender without being unfair. In this book we call all babies 'he'. They aren't of course, although there are a few more male than female babies born. More importantly, it makes it easier for the reader to sort out to whom a pronoun refers when both baby and mother are referred to in the same sentence.

We also assume that babies have two parents who live together and are married. Obviously this is not always true but the use of the term 'husband' makes writing (and reading) easier by cutting down on all the terms which otherwise have to be used to describe fathers, many of which are contrived and stilted. There is another reason too. We don't use the term 'your baby's father' all the time because fathers, like mothers, are other things as well as parents. Being a father is not the only social role they have. Indeed, that is one of the points we want to make. *Parents should not give so much of their lives away to their babies that there is nothing left of themselves.* If they do, all their emotional investment is in their children and they have nothing for each other and nothing to respect in themselves. Parents with empty marriages and low self-esteem live vicariously through their children. Instead of being stimulated and fulfilled through their own activities and experiences, they obtain such satisfactions primarily from their children's achievements. This is bad news for the children who have to satisfy their parents at the expense of their own individual development. Quite inappropriately these children come to feel responsible for their parents' state of mind. Later in life, and somewhat surprisingly, they will respect their parents less. Adolescents in particular will respond to parents whom they have seen to be in control of their own lives – those who have had and continue to have a range of interests and experiences beyond childcare. Good parents are more than merely parents.

Between us we have looked after or come to know professionally over 4,000 women with new babies, and what is so striking is the way in which the same problems and issues keep coming up. This means that we have been asked for a great deal of advice. With increasing experience we have found out what is important, what usually works and what doesn't.

Advice leads to the acquisition of knowledge and skills which are part of a new social role, in this case becoming a parent. For that reason there are some sections which deal with basic skills in looking after a tiny baby. Otherwise we have tried to keep the new mother in focus and urge her to do the same for herself. The final result is this short book which is meant to be practical, useful, and to place the new parents alongside the baby at the centre of things.

STAGE 1

Thinking ahead

1

Thinking ahead

This first section is best read when you are in the early stages of your pregnancy. You already have your baby but he is inside you. You are already looking after him but it doesn't take much conscious activity on your part. Babycare in pregnancy is on automatic pilot.

Yet when you give birth and your baby starts to live outside your body, you are going to have to do things actively in order to look after him. Like it or not, you will have to reorganise your life so that you can do this. This will be a bit of a shock to the system. But you can manage it, like you can manage so many other things, by some thinking ahead. Of course, you are already doing this but it may be little more than pleasant daydreaming. A small amount of planning can transform this into really useful mental activity.

One of the differences between competent parents and others is the extent to which they can be pro-active. Competent parents plan ahead and take the initiative rather than yield passively to a situation which then takes them over. Planning for life as a new parent is quite easy and it is rewarding. The curious thing is how few future parents think it necessary. The following sections explain things further.

2

It's not going to change my life! (Or is it?)

You might, quite reasonably, ask how something so small and helpless as a baby could manage to change *your* life? Why can't you carry on with your own existence and cope with looking after a baby – just like you have coped with so many other things?

When you become a parent for the first time, the world changes. Having a baby is even more of a life change than getting married – the other big commitment you make to sharing your life permanently with someone. Just like a husband, a baby makes demands on your time, forces his way into your affections and, yes, will be (even more) dependent. The phrase 'makes demands on your time' trips past quickly because it is a cliché, but this is exactly what happens – babies *demand*. They won't take no for an answer, even if you think you can teach them who's boss. And they take up a lot of time.

Any career woman with spirit will probably say that babies can be managed like anyone else. You can always go back to work and fax the nanny a few instructions, send the baby off to a day nursery by courier, arrange to be paged if it's time for a feed and so forth. Absolutely right in some senses – motherhood shouldn't take over the whole of a woman's life, and it needn't so long as you plan ahead. But part of planning and preparation is accepting that you will have little freedom of choice for the first few months. Your baby will be in charge. The balance of power shifts back towards you as your baby grows. In the beginning, though, his demands and his helplessness will pull you into a new phase of your life. You become a mother as well as everything else that you are.

What makes a baby so powerful that he will change your life for you? Part of this is the power of his sheer helplessness. He demands to be looked after because it is so obvious that he can't do much for himself. Babies have a well-developed capacity to elicit good parenting in order to survive. They have to make sure someone looks after them. They can't exist on their own and won't be able to for another dozen or so years.

Not that this is the whole story by any means. Looks count. There is something about babies that everyone finds attractive. In one study, university students (who have less to do with babies than virtually anyone else) were asked to rate pictures of babies' faces for attractiveness. They were shown various drawings and asked to choose the cutest. The one chosen by an overwhelming majority was the one which conformed most closely to a real baby's features. Like all babies, it had a round face with chubby cheeks and big black pupils to its eyes. Some students cut the picture out and pinned it on their wall. It had massive emotional appeal. It demanded attention.

A baby has the knack of ensuring that you get hooked on him, he makes you fall in love with him. Before you are pregnant, babies probably seem quite nice but rather less than wonderful. However, when you have your own he will quite simply bowl you over. He will make you want to pick him up, cuddle him, love him and he will plant roots in your heart and mind. That is how he ensures his own survival. It is also a way of making things easy and enjoyable for you.

Quite apart from the helplessness and the looks, there is also something special about your own baby. He is individual, unique, special and precious. It is not just that he has the equipment selected by evolution to ensure his survival by eliciting caring responses from adults, he forms a unique relationship with you. He is not just any young baby, he is yours and you are his. There is a special relationship which develops between the two of you.

For some mothers this is easy. From the moment of birth or from months beforehand they are in love with their baby. For quite a number of others, such feelings take some time to grow and there is no instant 'bonding' – something which is perfectly normal and we will return to. Do not panic that you may be the only woman who will not fall in love with her baby – he will make sure that you do eventually.

All this does not stem from the practicalities of having to look after him. Even if you have a full-time nanny, you will find that your baby will occupy a staggering amount of your thoughts and emotional energy because you will constantly think and perhaps worry about him. If he needs you he will cry, something which it is impossible to dismiss. You may be able to ignore the crying of other people's babies but not your own. He will sometimes make you feel as helpless as he does. Life honestly won't be the same as it was before.

All this is very difficult for many women with exciting

jobs, careers or an established lifestyle who are understandably determined to have their baby and carry on as they were before. 'It's not going to change my life,' they say. Their husbands will often take the same view – surely it is possible to get a baby into a routine and organise him in the same way that you have been able to do with other aspects of your life? However, babies have a powerful effect on the people around them, forcing themselves on to centre stage as far as attention goes, dominating their parents' emotions and making sure that the world revolves round them. Although they often do this in a way which is enjoyable, they have attributes which make sure that others will care for them and help them develop. By being attractive and lovable, they make sure that they are affectionately cared for. Ultimately what it means is that babies change people: they make it impossible for their parents to remain the people they used to be.

There are two aspects to the whole process which might be worth thinking about. Firstly, your place in the world changes – you take on a new role. You become a mother. This is quite different from what happens to you when you acquire a puppy. Becoming a parent is something which changes how you think, how you feel, what you do and how other people see you. Putting things the other way round, it is a curious reflection that the English language doesn't have a single noun for a person or couple who don't have children. When you have a child of your own you acquire a new part to your personality. In formal sociological terms it is known as a role transition – moving into parenthood.

Secondly, you will discover that your baby has an effect on you which continues throughout childhood and beyond. It isn't just the case that you will bring him up; he will also bring out aspects of you which might not otherwise have happened if he had not been there. *Children bring up parents as well as parents bring up children.* By their very existence they encourage their parents to learn about a new universe of child-related topics – toys, schools or childhood illnesses – which most adults would not otherwise bother with. They elicit new emotions from parents such as pride at their achievements and they make sure that their parents acquire new skills such as changing nappies or playing computer games.

You can, of course, move into the state of parenthood without giving it much thought – after all, most people do. What many pregnant women and their husbands do is focus all their attention on the forthcoming labour, culminating in the actual birth as the finale, without giving much thought to life with the baby afterwards. Sometimes they actively prevent themselves from thinking too much about life after birth because they worry that their baby may not turn out to be healthy. Quite a few people shut out of their minds the thoughts about what having a baby might entail. Better not to think about it until you have to, they say. Things will work out. Everyone copes in the end.

But sometimes they don't cope very well and become demoralised and exhausted. Certainly you will survive if you don't plan, but at a cost to yourself and your marriage. It would seem sensible to be reasonably prepared beforehand so that you can manage things and be more in charge. By making a small number of plans and arrangements you are less likely to be knocked sideways by the change in your life. Even so, many (probably most) women will find themselves thrown seriously off balance. The arrangements and plans made beforehand will enable you to regain your equilibrium sooner and thus survive the process much better. Most importantly, you are then much more likely to enjoy it.

Similarly, you will cope more positively with having a baby and becoming a parent by having realistic expectations and a little insight. The whole business can, after all, be deeply satisfying. Planning ahead and keeping a sense of proportion (and humour) will help avoid the pitfalls such as panic, feeling overwhelmed or losing your confidence, all of which are the common side-effects of becoming a parent for the first time. You can't anticipate everything but you can begin to think practically about how you and your baby will be after the delivery. This is something which is more than daydreaming and which means doing some active thinking ahead and making plans accordingly.

Some people get sentimental and say they would rather not plan anything but prefer to let it happen 'naturally' so their response is spontaneous. Certainly babies will help elicit this response but they may overstate their case. They can present such a demand on you that you become overwhelmed by parenthood. The paradox is that you can only allow yourself to be genuinely spontaneous *if you are in charge of your life*, otherwise the number of things you can do spontaneously is limited. If you are feeling drained, the only thing you can do spontaneously is fall asleep. If you lose your confidence you will find yourself having a good spontaneous worry.

Having a small baby can drain you and sap your self-confidence. Does your baby really want you to be tired, irritable and feeling useless? Does he want to hear you and your husband snapping at each other? Is this the natural state of affairs you wanted? No, it isn't, and it is no good for your baby either. While everyone with a baby gets ratty and rattled at some time, it can be cut to a minimum. It is also possible to enjoy your baby rather than experience him only as overwhelming. In order to make this happen, we argue, on the basis of all the new mothers we have known, that it is vastly better to manage things pro-actively – which means forethought and planning. That is what this book is all about.

3

Work and when to stop it

Many pregnant women fall into an understandable trap. They think that the right thing to do is to work up to the very last moment so they can then have the maximum amount of time off after the birth to spend with their baby. While that is perfectly true in terms of time allowed for maternity leave, it is not usually the best plan for you or your baby's health. Even worse, it can be justified by inappropriately tough-minded values ('I'm going to work up to the last possible minute, I can cope with having it under a hedge if necessary') or mistaken psychology ('I'm going to work until the head crowns because I will then have all my maternity leave to spend with my baby afterwards so that I can really bond to him').

If you have a set number of weeks for maternity leave, give up work earlier and return earlier. We suggest you stop work by 34 weeks. The reasons for this are as follows:

- Firstly, your baby is already there. It is just that he is inside you. Until he is born, he it totally dependent upon the physical care which only you can provide.

After he is born, other people can help, but beforehand they can't. You can, by what you do, affect the quality of the physical care you provide for him even before he is born. Take the issue of having a rest for instance. During the last three months of pregnancy it becomes progressively more important that you have a rest lying down sometime during the day because this maximises the blood flow to the placenta and so to your baby. Few jobs will allow you to do this. Apart from the direct benefit to your baby, daily rest is also an important preventive measure in avoiding high blood pressure which is a hazard for your pregnancy (and in any case the treatment for raised blood pressure is enforced bed rest, sometimes in hospital). Work nearly always gets in the way of adequate rest. That's why it's called work.

- Secondly, giving up paid work and beginning to spend all your time at home is a major change in lifestyle. It is what psychologists call a life event, something which, when it happens to you, can make you emotionally vulnerable. Social scientists would take a different perspective and refer to a role transition as you move from being a worker to (face it) a housewife. Both groups draw the same conclusion: believe it or not, stopping work – even if you are planning to return – can be quite stressful. It can be the opposite of beginning to take things easy and it takes time to adjust to. You find yourself on your own for much of the day and have to restructure your time. The longer you have worked, the more unsettling it is. You may miss your routines, your peer group and the general stimulation. It isn't necessary to be a workaholic to feel uneasy or even anxious on stopping work.
- If giving up work is one life event, having a baby is yet another one and imposes a further role transition as

you become a parent. You honestly don't want to have to cope with two life events or role transitions at once. Ideally, they need to be separated by about six weeks. It is also worth bearing in mind that it is as normal for babies to arrive two weeks early as it is for them to arrive two weeks late. A small proportion of babies (7 per cent) will arrive three or four weeks early, which means that the six weeks you may have allocated for preparation and adjustment becomes two or three weeks, which is simply not long enough. (On the subject of early labour, not working right up to the end means that it is less likely your waters will break in the office.)

- Thirdly, it pays to get into some good habits before the birth so that you don't have to struggle to establish them after. Having an afternoon rest is one such habit. It is important for the health of your baby before he is born and it is important for your health afterwards. *Sleep deprivation is always more of a problem for new mothers than any of them expect.* If you have established a habit of a nap during the day and can then continue with it after your baby is born, you will be able to recuperate more quickly. Otherwise it will take several weeks to establish a new habit of a siesta. You can't learn to sleep at home in the afternoon and carry on with work at the same time.
- Fourthly, things happen to your energy, your mood and your thought processes in late pregnancy, after about 34 weeks. Sometimes it happens earlier. Indeed, for some, post-coital drowsiness never quite wears off. If you have a high-powered job, the odds are that you will ordinarily be hyped-up in order to do it well. Yet the vast majority of women in late pregnancy experience an inevitable slowing of their activity and their thinking

whether they want this or not. At the same time, it is common for women in the later stages of pregnancy to find themselves less able to concentrate, more emotional, less decisive, more irritable, tiring more easily and less able to assert themselves. Do take seriously the possibility that even you will experience some of this. Like PMT, it can apply to the strongest-willed and most capable people.

- At the same time as all this, broody thoughts about her forthcoming baby and babies in general begin to intrude and preoccupy the mother-to-be during the last six weeks of pregnancy. The most unlikely women may find themselves peering into other people's prams and becoming riveted by the Mothercare catalogue. This is a well-recognised phenomenon known as *primary maternal preoccupation*. It helps the woman prepare psychologically for looking after a dependent baby and the forthcoming role transition into new motherhood. It doesn't, however, tend to help you manage high-powered work. Neither slowing of thought nor maternal preoccupations will help you with a demanding job.
- Finally, it is very difficult for women to anticipate the physical tiredness that many of them will experience in late pregnancy. Simple activities, such as getting in and out of a car or picking things up from the floor, require enormous effort, especially if you have put on extra weight. If you work up to the last moment and exhaust yourself as a consequence, the quality of time you can offer your baby after the birth may be compromised simply because you will be drained and irritable. In childcare, what counts is the quality of time spent with children, not its quantity. It is better to spend brief amounts of quality time with your baby in which you

can give him undivided, generous, responsive attention rather than weeks on end of short-temperedness while you blame him for not letting you rest.

The best advice, provided you have some say in the matter, is to stop work by 34 weeks, even if you are planning to return to work after the birth. Try to use your maternity leave to give up work sooner and return to it earlier – it is not a disaster if you can't but it is better if you can. Your return to work should be between six weeks and six months after your baby's birth. (See Stage 5.)

HOLIDAYS

If you are planning a holiday abroad, you will not be allowed to fly after you are 36 weeks' pregnant. Between 28 and 36 weeks you will need a letter from your doctor, stating your expected dates of delivery (EDD) and level of fitness.

THINKING AHEAD ABOUT MONEY

One of the worst aspects of new motherhood for women with a career is loss of financial independence – be it temporary or permanent. If you are not going to return to work after your baby is born, sort out the future family finances with your husband early in pregnancy. This means you and your husband should decide whether you are going to have a joint account and/or a house-keeping allowance and how much you will need or you both can afford. Thoroughly capable women often feel helpless soon after having a baby. If you are feeling rather useless at that time you will not want to experience the further humiliation of continually having to ask your husband for money.

While on the subject of money, bear in mind that when you return to work your career progress may be compromised by the demands and considerable expenses of childcare. Aim simply to stay where you are on the career ladder rather than climb it further during your child's early years. Plan to maintain your earning capacity, not advance it. You may well do better than this but don't expect to. If you set your sights too high there is the risk that you may be disappointed. It would be more realistic to expect simply to keep your feet on the same rung as before and break even financially.

4

Antenatal classes

It is not quite as easy as it might seem to make straightforward points about antenatal classes. At one level they are obviously a good thing, yet what one course offers is quite likely to be different from another. If you are in the fortunate position of being able to choose which ones to go to (which probably only applies to people living in cities or large towns) then it pays to think about what they can do for you. Then, by asking around, you can find out what goes on and choose accordingly. Hospital classes are generally sound, though sometimes unexciting, and have the advantage of familiarising you with names, faces and the building where it's ultimately all going to happen.

The main point of antenatal classes is to educate people so that they are not frightened during labour. They will also explain how to recognise the onset of labour; when to go into hospital; what is going to happen there; the language used by health professionals to describe the processes involved in childbirth; how to manage contractions; what forms of pain relief are available; and how to help the midwives deliver your baby. Whatever else the classes do, they must cover this ground.

Some classes go further. The better ones provide a framework for understanding the process of birth in terms of female anatomy and physiology. They will also explain when and why medical interventions may be necessary. The best take the whole process beyond the birth (which of course is not the finale) and discuss current feeding techniques and basic babycare as well as the potential problems that are likely to arise when caring for a new baby.

Classes which are exercise-based are an extension of the above and not a substitute for them. They are not strictly necessary but a number of mothers enjoy them. Check that the class leader has herself been on a specific course on the supervision of exercises during pregnancy. The ligaments which stabilise joints become looser during pregnancy. This, coupled with stretched abdominal muscles which are less able to stabilise the lower spine, means that pregnant women need careful supervision during exercise classes to ensure that they do not strain their back or damage (rather than strengthen!) their abdominal muscles. It is not quite so much that there are certain exercises to avoid during pregnancy but the need for intensive exercise to be supervised by an expert.

There are classes which concentrate solely on preparation for 'natural' childbirth or on idiosyncratic techniques for giving birth. These ultimately hinge upon you having a short, straightforward labour – something which is difficult to predict with certainty, particularly because it depends largely on the position of your baby just before birth and the shape of your pelvic bones. With this in mind, beware of classes which take an ideological stance, which insist that it is best to deliver in a particular position or place, and which oppose all forms of pain control or are anti-midwife or anti-obstetrician. Be very wary of classes which assume you can choose the kind of labour you will have.

Left to nature, the vast majority of women (87 per cent) will have a labour which does not require medical intervention. This is the 'natural' birth that can make those fortunate enough to experience it feel proud that they have done it all on their own without medical intervention. It is an experience that they will understandably feel satisfied about. The difficulty is that, particularly when it is your first baby, no one, not even your doctor or midwife, can be absolutely definite that you will have a natural birth until the very last minute. It is not something that you, or anyone else, can make happen with any certainty because it hinges upon your baby and your pelvis. You may, at the start of your pregnancy, be determined to have a natural birth. The chances are that you will but actually you haven't the choice; there is nothing you or your classes can do to ensure it. If anything it is your baby's choice and even he can't have it all his own way if your pelvis is a difficult size or shape for his purposes. He may also decide to be born in an awkward way and you can't change that. Bear in mind that childbirth used to be inevitably 'natural', and was one of the commonest causes of death for women and their babies. It isn't nowadays because of advances in obstetric techniques but that doesn't mean that, left to nature, anything has changed. You can prepare for a 'natural' birth and you may hope to have one but you can't make it happen if it isn't going to.

Nor does it matter as far as your baby is concerned. Apart from the very few babies who have been snatched from the jaws of death, babies born with medical help are ultimately no different from those who were born 'naturally'. In later life, people who were born 'naturally' do not differ from those whose birth required obstetric intervention or whose mothers were given pain relief. Some mothers are understandably, though inappropriately, concerned that in order to give their babies a 'perfect start' they have to have a 'natural' birth. Honestly, there is no factual basis for this.

Thus if you happen to fall into the 13 per cent who can't have a baby without medical help, you may feel you have in some way failed, especially if you have been to the type of class which leads you to anticipate a brief, uncomplicated birth or which implies that it is up to you. Actually, *labour isn't one of those things which you can pass or fail.* No amount of special diets, exercises or breathing practice will ultimately affect the shape of your pelvis or the position of your baby at the onset of labour. Having a rigid idea of how you are going to have your baby, whether as an idea in your head or as a written birth plan, is risky because at the end of the day nature may not necessarily let you have your own way, even when the hospital backs your ideas to begin with. You can be prepared but you cannot control.

This is another example of the way in which your baby has a say in things right from the start. The baby has some influence over his own delivery. You can no more plan exactly how you will give birth than dictate that you are going to have a fair-haired baby girl. Good classes recognise that it is in your interest to have realistic expectations, which means you will be prepared for a range of eventualities.

In the long run the most important thing is that you have a healthy baby and that you can look back on your delivery with positive feelings, not feeling that you have 'failed' some sort of test because you had to have an episiotomy, an epidural, forceps or a Caesarean section. If you are led to believe that you are inadequate because you couldn't 'achieve' a 'natural' birth, you will spend the first few days after the birth thinking backwards about what went 'wrong' rather than enjoying your new baby. This is very bad news for you and we have seen wholly avoidable postnatal depressions triggered by such feelings of disappointment and failure.

Although there are some sets of classes which are primarily for couples, there is no firm principle that states that these are 'better'. Dragging unwilling fathers-to-be along to them can be disruptive for the whole group and the sort of detail which many women welcome is not necessarily appealing to men. Some men are riveted by the whole process of pregnancy and birth, some are not. In the long run, either sort of man can be a totally competent husband and father. Good courses will have a fathers' evening but to go beyond this is a matter of personal choice, not an inevitable improvement.

Of course, you can educate yourself by reading books, or you may be medically trained and feel that you don't need antenatal classes. However, your own pregnancy is special. Having your own baby, rather than seeing or helping with somebody else's delivery, is a totally different experience. Techniques may have changed since the books you choose to read were written or since you were trained, and a good class teacher will be up-to-date with local practice. In any case, participating actively in discussions in antenatal classes helps you to start to plan ahead more practically than mere daydreaming.

One of the most remarkable things about parents with children is that they tend to sort themselves into groups according to the age of their eldest child. In a sense, the child chooses their social group for them. Parents of young children often feel they have less in common with parents of older children and vice versa. To a certain extent this is because talking to each other about their own children is something that people do a great deal, and it helps if the children under discussion are at a similar stage of development or schooling. As an extension of this, it also helps parents if they can learn from other parents what baby equipment works well, what helps small children go to sleep, which toys are popular, or which schools are best. In other words, having a group of parents with similar-aged children is a resource for all of them which provides information and support.

For many parents, the origin of such a group was their antenatal class. With this in mind, it pays to weigh up whether the people who typically attend a particular course of classes are those with whom you will feel comfortable.

5

Exercise during pregnancy

This heading could equally well read 'exercise for the childbearing year' since the types of exercises that you do when pregnant can have important benefits for your body after childbirth.

If you have been exercising regularly before you became pregnant, you will probably want to continue during your pregnancy. This is fine so long as you feel comfortable during the exercise, though you should reduce the amount you do. Your *total weekly exercise time* should tot up to about *two-thirds* of what you were doing before pregnancy. If you do the same amount of exercise during pregnancy as you were doing before, there is a risk that your blood supply will be diverted from the placenta, which is obviously not in the interests of your baby. The same general principle applies to exercise classes: you can continue them as long as your teacher knows you are pregnant and modifies active abdominal muscle exercises to take your pregnancy into account.

If you are a person who normally takes no exercise but you feel pregnancy is the time to begin, be clear what the benefits are. Your primary reason for exercising is to feel better in yourself through general fitness, not because it makes you more likely to have a straightforward labour. In spite of what you may be led to believe, there is *absolutely no evidence* that physical fitness has any effect at all on the length and type of labour you will experience. However, women who are reasonably fit will have more stamina for a long labour. Fit women also tend to recover physically and heal more quickly following childbirth.

You don't have to join an exercise class to exercise. In fact an amateur class with a hyperactive leader should be avoided because inappropriately vigorous 'impact' exercises can strain ligaments already loosened during pregnancy, quite apart from the effects on blood flow mentioned above. In general terms, swimming (one to three times a week for up to half an hour at a time) is an ideal exercise for pregnant women so long as they avoid arching their lower back excessively during breast stroke. If you find your back is aching after swimming, change your stroke.

There are two groups of muscles that literally take most of the strain during pregnancy – the pelvic floor muscles and the abdominals (tummy muscles). It is worth giving these specific attention during pregnancy because of their importance to you afterwards. Look after these muscle groups as well as you can – they will, after all, be with you long after your baby has grown up and left home.

PELVIC FLOOR MUSCLES

The pelvic floor is the name given to the muscles that are attached to the bottom of the pelvis. They are responsible for supporting the organs of the pelvis (lower bowel, uterus and bladder) while allowing three openings – the anus, the vagina and the urethra (through which you pee) – to pass through the muscular floor to the outside.

If these muscles weaken and sag, they can no longer support the contents of the pelvis properly and will not help the openings to close off properly, causing embarrassing problems. The commonest of these is stress incontinence – inadvertently wetting yourself when coughing or laughing – while the more serious complications include prolapse which is when the uterus starts to sag down through the vagina, or the vaginal walls collapse under pressure from a full bladder or bowel.

The weight of a pregnant uterus and the way in which the pelvic floor must stretch to allow a baby through the vaginal opening during childbirth mean that the whole business of having a baby puts the pelvic floor muscles under enormous strain. Most women will find their pelvic floor muscles bruised and sore after birth – some will find they have a crutch full of stitches, especially following a forceps delivery. Whatever state you find yourself in after the birth (and even after a Caesarean birth), you will need to perform pelvic floor exercises as soon as possible in order to help these muscles recover quickly and restore their strength. The process, however, is best started well before the postnatal period. Through exercising your pelvic floor during pregnancy, you are keeping as much tone in the muscles as possible and getting yourself 'programmed' so that exercising them regularly becomes second nature.

By doing this, you will have established an important habit well before the postnatal period which is when you will need to rehabilitate them actively. This is crucial future insurance to prevent prolapse or stress incontinence later in life (there are few things more ageing than wet knickers). It follows that the pelvic floor muscles are the only group of muscles in the body which really do need to be exercised religiously throughout pregnancy.

HOW TO DO IT

The muscles of the pelvic floor are arranged in two layers. One layer is like a hammock or sling stretching across between the pubic bone at the front of your pelvis and the coccyx (tailbone) at the base of your spine. The second layer is composed of groups of circular muscle fibres around the openings of the anus, the vagina and the urethra. Thus, when you contract the pelvic floor muscles, two movements occur – you pull up the hammock muscle and at the same time you tighten up round each of the openings. Therefore, if you want to contract the pelvic floor fully, imagine that you need to prevent an accidental bowel movement, stop a tampon falling out, and have a full bladder but can't get to the loo – all at the same time. When

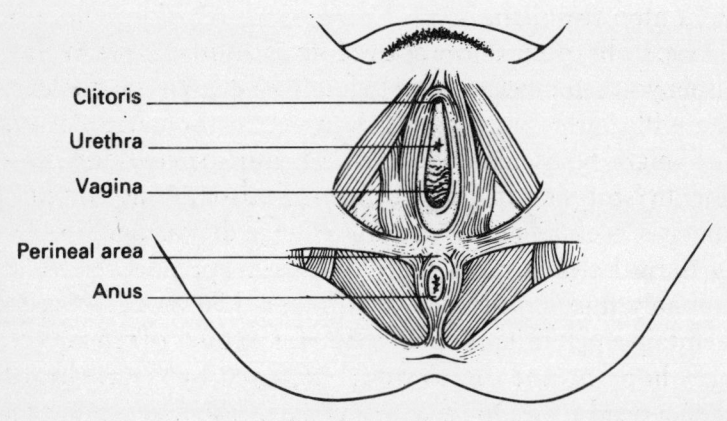

Figure 1 The pelvic floor muscles

you then relax your pelvic floor you should be aware of a slight 'dropping' feeling of the hammock muscle.

During pregnancy, start by pulling up the pelvic floor muscles as a whole group and then relax them, doing this in groups of five contractions at a time, at least five times a day. This means you will do at least 25 contractions a day. This should be done in any position – not just when you are sitting down. While you are contracting and relaxing your pelvic floor, other muscle groups should not be working as well. Try very hard to concentrate on contracting and relaxing your pelvic floor muscles separately from your tummy and buttock muscles which often try to contract at the same time. Most women find that learning to isolate their pelvic floor contractions in this way takes a bit of practice. Once you are able to carry out an isolated pelvic floor contraction with minimum effort, you can focus down and concentrate just on tightening the circular muscle around the vagina – the other muscles will work as well and that does not matter; it is the muscle around the vagina that is the one that will need the most concentrated work after the birth.

Hopefully, none of the above information is news to you. Either you are an old hand at pelvic floor exercises, or at least you will have started them during your antenatal classes. You might be accustomed to doing your pelvic floor exercises by stopping the flow of urine midstream as you pee. This is a useful way to teach non-pregnant women how to use the muscles correctly, but when you are pregnant you will probably find it depressingly difficult. Likewise, trying to maintain a pelvic floor contraction for a count of ten may be fairly hopeless and the 'elevator' exercise (if you have heard of it) a dead loss. Don't worry if this is the case – you will return to all these advanced tests and exercises after the baby has been born.

Don't be tempted to do hundreds of pelvic floor lifts on the same occasion and think that will see you through for the next few weeks. The circular muscles tire very quickly so after a few contractions they will work less effectively and the exercise loses its usefulness.

The best way of remembering to do pelvic floor exercises is whenever you are bored or slightly impatient (check-out queues in the supermarket, waiting at red traffic lights, in an antenatal clinic or sitting next to someone very tedious at a dinner party). What you need to do during pregnancy is to get into an automatic habit and 'programme' yourself to carry out the 25 lifts a day while being barely conscious of doing it.

Once you have had your baby, you will need to do around 50 lifts a day until you have a very strong pelvic floor again – possibly even better than it was before you became pregnant. Even after all this, wise women will continue to do ten lifts a day (still in groups of five) as a well-woman exercise throughout their lives, partly to guard against prolapse and stress incontinence, and partly (and no genius is required to realise this) because these muscles will play a major role in your future sex life.

YOUR BACK AND YOUR FRONT

Nobody wants backache and nobody wants a pot belly as well as a baby. The two are connected: both have to do with your back. Back care sounds boring and not everyone is fascinated by bones and muscles. But consider the following:

- 80 per cent of women suffer from back problems at some stage during their life.

- Nearly all of these women have children.
- Pregnancy softens the ligaments, which hold the joints in your back together.
- Carting a baby around, whether inside you or outside you, changes your posture.
- Altered posture puts a strain on your back.
- Being a parent means bending down a lot.

There is no need to panic that you are sentenced to back trouble just because you are pregnant. Avoiding back problems is (a) possible and (b) not too difficult. What you need is a piece of knowledge and the capacity to do something actively – just like so many things to do with becoming a competent parent.

The relevant piece of knowledge (and not many people know this) is that it is *weak tummy muscles*, not weak back muscles, which are generally responsible for low back strain. The active work is what you do to keep them in good shape during pregnancy. It is much easier to prevent backache than cure it. It also helps prevent you developing a pot belly afterwards.

All this needs some explanation. Abdominal (tummy) muscles form an elastic sheet under the skin. This sheet is fixed to your spine at the back, your ribs at the top and your pelvis at the bottom. It is rather like an old-fashioned corset and means that everything in your abdomen is held inside a tube with muscle at the front and sides and bony structures at the top, bottom and back.

At the front there are two long muscles overlying the sheet which run from the rib cage down to the brim of the pelvis. These are part of your total abdominal musculature and act like luggage straps. When they contract, they pull the front of your rib cage and the front of your pelvis closer together. Normally, all your abdominal muscles act

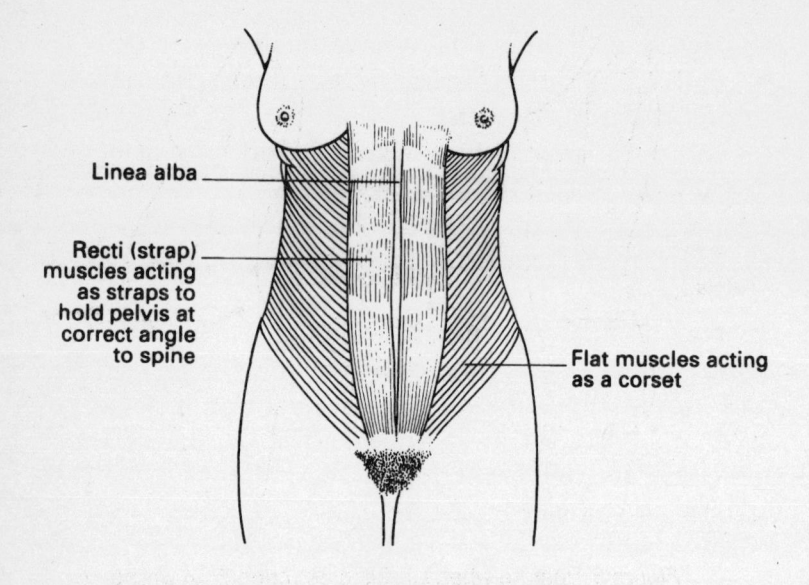

Figure 2 The abdominal muscles

together to brace themselves and form a tight wall. In doing so they protect the contents of your abdomen. They also, acting together with your buttock muscles, line your pelvis up correctly. However, by being stretched over your bulge they are weakened.

The pelvis is a bowl of bone at the bottom of your spine. It can tip forward like a bucket or wheelbarrow does when you are emptying one. Normally it is held by abdominal and buttock muscles at a shallow angle in relation to your back and your legs. This is *correct* pelvic tilt. When this tilt is at the correct angle, the muscle groups around the base of your spine are in balance and the hollow in the small of your back is limited.

When you are pregnant, three things happen:

EXERCISE DURING PREGNANCY

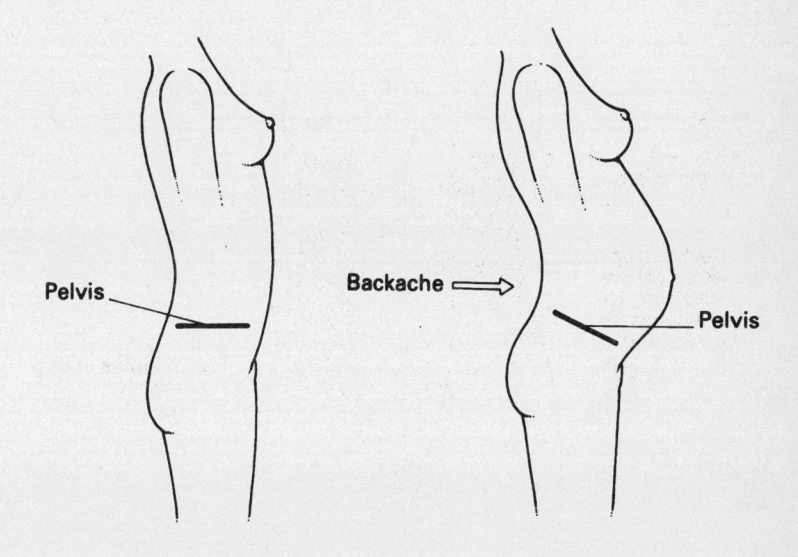

Figure 3 Posture when standing: (a) correct (b) wrong

- The heavy uterus sitting on your pelvis bulges forwards out of your lower abdomen. It can't bulge backwards because your spine is in the way.
- This large uterus stretches your front abdominal muscle wall so that these muscles are weakened.
- Your joints are looser because of hormonal action on the ligaments. Thus your back bends more readily.

This means that there is a powerful tendency for the uterus to slump forward, poorly restrained by the abdominal muscles. The pelvis tilts forward beyond its correct angle like a wheelbarrow overloaded at the front. This pulls the supple (and therefore vulnerable) lower back into an even hollower curve than normal.

To add to this strain on her back, the pregnant woman has to lean back when walking to avoid falling forward.

Her centre of gravity is so far forward she has to balance it by leaning back and carrying all before, so the hollow in her back increases yet more. Haven't you seen women standing like this and massaging their aching lower back?

What you need to do is maintain as good a tone as possible in your abdominal muscles. Keep them elastic. You don't want overstretched abdominal muscles because they have less elasticity and can't accommodate and restrain a growing uterus.

The key to well-toned elastic muscles is a secret exercise which you carry out while going about your ordinary life. Hold your tummy muscles in while walking and think 'tight tummy'. Make yourself look three months less pregnant than you actually are. Don't wear a girdle (unless a physiotherapist tells you to. She may if you are expecting twins, for instance). Don't wear high heels because they make you lean backwards to keep upright and this increases the hollow in your back.

Active strengthening exercises for abdominal muscles may be fine but no better than the one above. What you need to aim for is good muscle tone, not powerful muscle strength. You want an elastic abdominal wall, not a rigid iron one.

All this is easier for large women, for tall women and for those who are not carrying a baby which is lying awkwardly. The petite woman with a baby who engages late or not at all has more of an overspill problem. She will need to think 'tight tummy' more of the time.

If you notice that the strap muscles which run up and down your front (the recti) balloon out over your pregnancy bump when you sit up in the bath, stop doing any full sit-up exercises. You are putting too much strain on the strap muscles and overstretching them. Watch out for other times when you might strain them and develop habits

EXERCISE DURING PREGNANCY

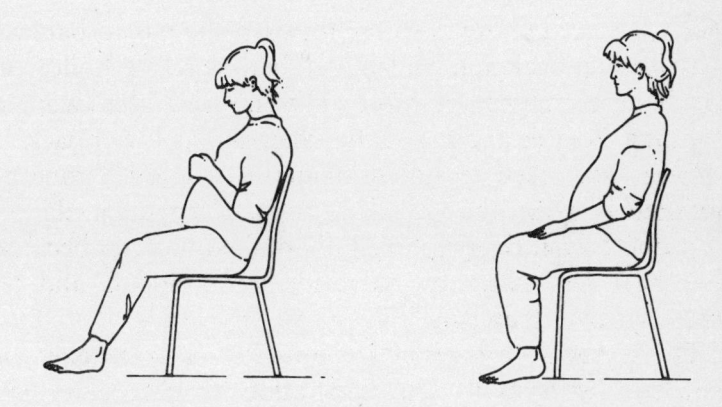

Figure 4 Posture when sitting: (a) wrong (b) correct

which protect them. For instance, when you get out of bed, roll over onto your side (keeping your knees together) and let your arms rather than your tummy muscles get you upright. Once muscles have overstretched they lose their elasticity. An overstretched spring is feeble.

When you are sitting, make sure your bottom is well back in the chair so that your lower back has some support from the chair back. If you are going to spend any time at a desk or in front of a computer, the seat of a chair should be low enough for you to rest your feet flat on the floor. The sort of chair which has no back but pads on which you kneel while sitting is fine for desk work but tends to be uncomfortable for sitting when relaxing. In any case try to shift your posture every so often and avoid sitting in any position for more than two hours continuously.

Be very careful when lifting. Always bend your knees and keep your back straight to pick something up – even a tissue from the floor. In theory you can squat, but this is not exactly practical in a short skirt in the office. In any case,

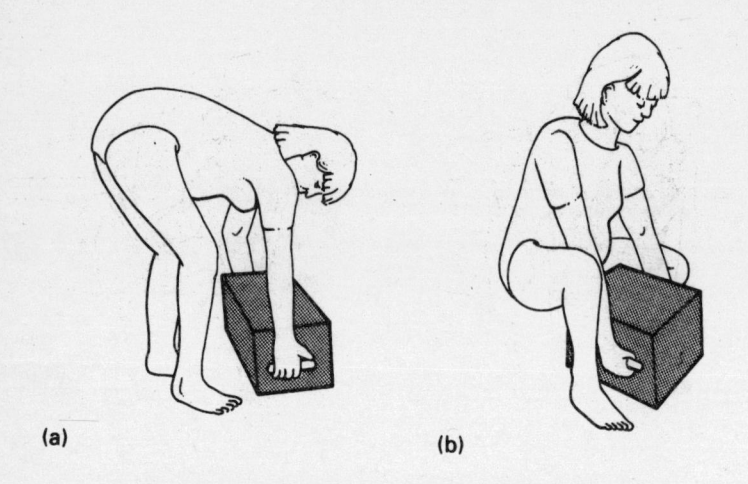

Figure 5 Bending down and lifting: (a) wrong (b) correct

most women who are heavily pregnant will find it easier to go down onto one knee. Being careful to keep a straight back is a rule which applies to unloading or feeding a washing machine or delving into a low cupboard in the kitchen.

A dishwasher is an ergonomic disaster area during pregnancy and the three months after delivery. If it is placed on the floor, it is almost impossible to load and unload without putting a strain on your lower back, so make sure your husband takes on dishwasher duties. Actually, a dishwasher can easily be mounted on a low cupboard so that it opens just below waist height but it seems that fitted kitchens are all designed by men or women who haven't had children. It is apparently quite ordinary to mount an oven at waist height but the idea of doing much the same with a dishwasher hasn't caught on (and, yes, we have suggested it to a kitchen unit manufacturer but with zero result).

EXERCISE DURING PREGNANCY

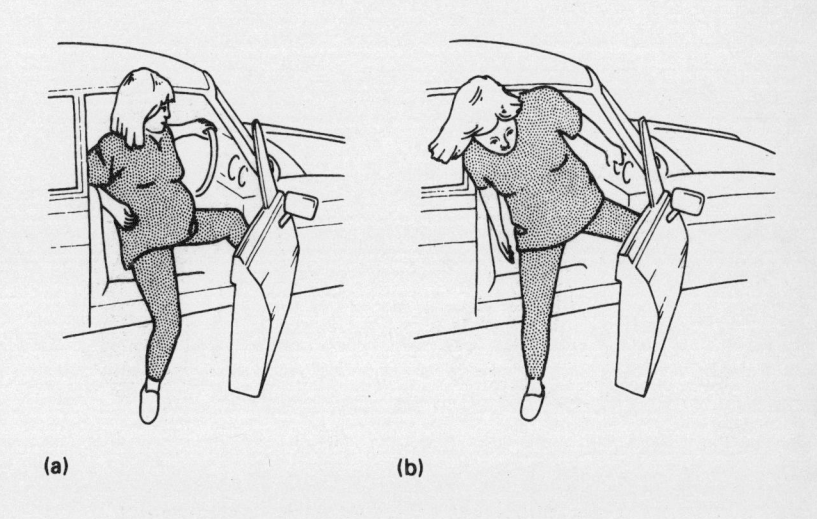

(a)　　　　　　　　　(b)

Figure 6a Getting into and out of a car the *wrong* way

Cars can present problems too. If you are driving, shift the seat closer to the steering wheel than you have it normally so that you operate the clutch using just your foot and ankle, rather than through your hip with a straight leg. Get in and out as though you are at a film premiere and being filmed yourself. To get in, back down bottom first, then swing both your legs in one after the other (smiling sweetly). Getting out means the reverse: swing one leg out, then the other, then lean forward, out and stand up. All this will not only help your back but prevent straining the pelvis. Unfortunately it is helped by having a sensible (boring) car – not too low and one which, for later uses, has four doors and in which you can eventually fit a baby/toddler seat.

Even when you get into bed, continue to think about your posture. On getting into bed you should lie on your back with your knees bent and actively pull your tummy

(a)

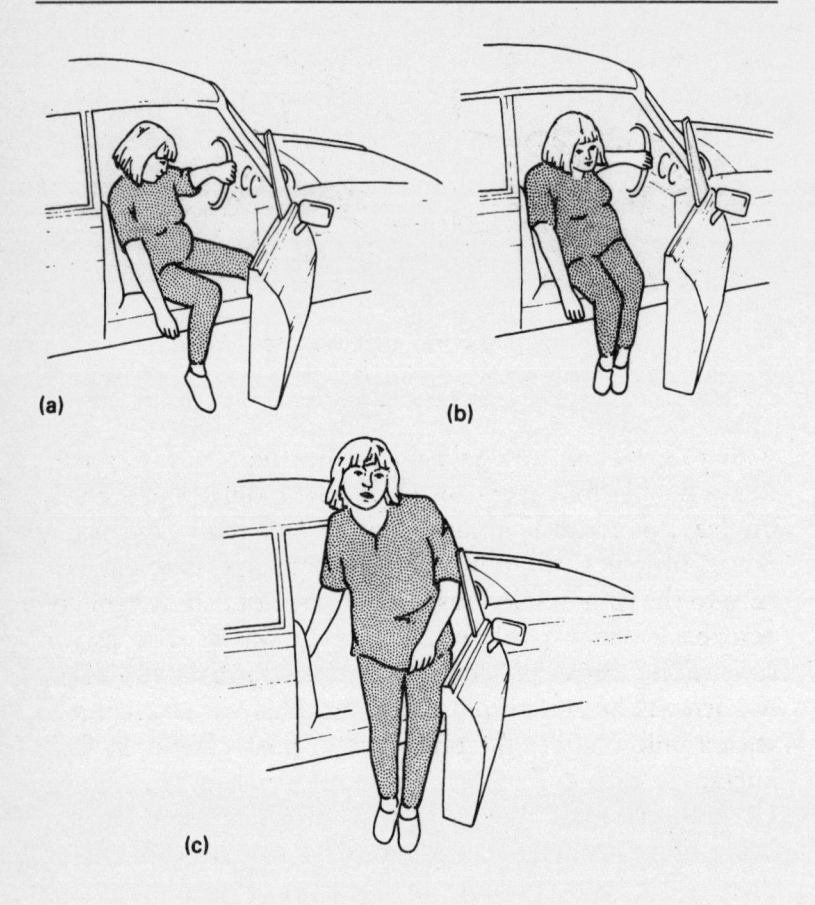

(b)

(c)

Figure 6b Getting into and out of a car the *correct* way

muscles in to flatten the small of the back against the mattress (pelvic tilt exercise) three times (see page 43). This is a comfortable exercise which corrects the tendency of your back muscles to shorten and pull your back into a bow.

If you are somebody who goes to sleep on your back you may find it more comfortable to put two pillows under

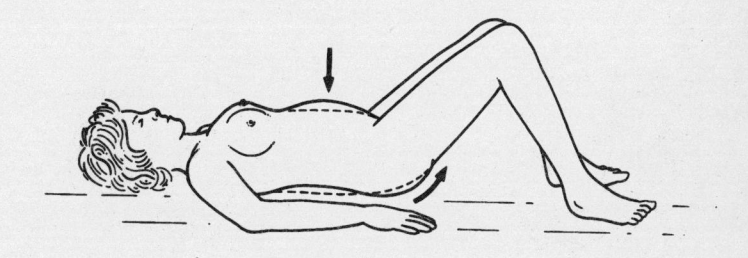

Figure 7 Pelvic tilt exercise

your thighs close up against your bottom. As it happens, many people find lying on their backs during pregnancy unpleasant because it makes them feel faint (the heavy uterus obstructs the flow of blood through the great vein next to the spine). Obviously if you are not comfortable on your back you will roll over onto your side as soon as you have done three pelvic tilts. In late pregnancy, many women will be at their most comfortable lying on their side with a pillow under the bump and a pillow between their knees.

6

Thinking ahead about yourself as a new mother

Try to visualise yourself with your baby practically and realistically. There are a large number of positive and pleasurable things about a new baby: you will love him (in spite of your worst fears that you will prove to be the one woman in the world who will not) and he will love you. He will provide you with one of the closest and most rewarding relationships you will ever experience, and as he grows and develops your sense of excitement and achievement will be extraordinary.

ORGANISING SUPPORT

As well as the good news, there are some tricky bits which you can manage better if you anticipate them. For instance, you are going to be very tired. Physically you will have gone through the exhausting process of labour which will be followed by a seemingly interminable period of broken nights. Most babies do not sleep through the night for the *first three months*. Your world will centre around caring for your baby and many of the exciting things you do now which stimulate you (such as going out with friends) will be more difficult to arrange. You will fall into step with your baby's demands and routines and find it impossible to ignore his calls on your time. Having spent much of the pregnancy secretly worrying as to whether their babies will be all right, many women find it hard to relax, even when they have a perfect baby. They continue to nurture another secret worry as to whether their baby will *remain* all right. This leads to emotional fatigue as well as physical tiredness. You may well find yourself simultaneously exhilarated and exhausted during the first few weeks.

As an extension of this, you will not exactly have time on your hands. Looking after a new baby is very much a full-time job. Your timetable will not allow you much opportunity for shopping, cooking, entertaining or, indeed, resting when you feel like it.

Your emotional life will change. Most women find that in the first few weeks after childbirth they are more emotionally volatile and dependent on their husband and others than before. They laugh, cry and fret more readily than they usually do. This is especially marked during the 'baby blues' phase a few days after the birth but frequently persists at a lower degree of intensity for several weeks after returning home. It is almost certainly caused by hormonal changes. Some women go into manic overdrive for a few days after returning home and exhaust themselves. This emotional turbulence is likely to be coupled with a difficulty in making decisions. All this can come as a bit of a shock to competent, highly organised career women (and to their husbands).

At the same time, it is a very common experience for new

mothers to find themselves worrying about all sorts of minor things to do with their babies, something which can make them feel that they have lost their sense of proportion and judgement. This contributes to a crisis of self-confidence which occurs in just about everyone – including new mothers who happen to be paediatricians.

What this means is that, once you come home after the birth, you are going to need some practical and emotional support if you are to enjoy your new baby fully. If someone else is helping you with the practicalities and minor hassles as well as boosting your confidence (should it start to flag), then you have more space in your life for the positive aspects of looking after a new baby.

For a start, your husband should plan his work schedule so that he is available to be with you not just while you are in labour but when you come home too. This planning is in itself quite difficult, as expected dates of delivery (EDDs) are informed guesses and as mentioned before, it is not uncommon for babies to be born two weeks either side of their due date. There isn't actually much point in your husband taking time off work while you are in hospital, but he will need to be free in the early evenings to visit you! You will also be dependent on him to do any shopping you might need (mainly food) and to wash and return your nighties and towels. Check that he knows how to operate the washing machine. Because you are used to coping well with things at home, you might be tempted to tell him that he shouldn't worry about taking time off and that you will manage without him if his work can't be shifted. Although this is generous and understanding of you, it is almost certainly not in either of your best interests.

Discuss with him and generally think hard about whether and when you should have your mother (or his mother) to stay. As a general rule it is better to stagger things. This means that the two of you can plan for your husband to take three or four days off when you come home. Then your mother or his can come and stay when he has gone back to work. It is difficult for everyone to balance things if you, the baby, your husband and your mother all establish themselves at home at the same time. Three generations coming simultaneously into a home where there has previously been one generation can be overwhelming. You, your baby and your husband need a few days at home together to settle down as a new family first. Capitalise on the fact that this is a good time.

If you are thinking of employing a maternity nurse to look after your baby, she will start as soon as you return home but there is still a clear role for your husband which is looking after *you*. You will need to interview and book her beforehand, of course. There are some issues about maternity nurses which are listed separately at the back of this book (see pages 211–14).

You won't have the time or the energy for cooking, so stock up your freezer beforehand with ready-prepared and instant meals. A trip to the supermarket accompanied by a tiny baby can be very anxiety provoking and needs to be avoided for as long as possible.

ORGANISING EVENTS AROUND THE BIRTH PERIOD

You may be faced with a two-week period of emptiness and anticipation after the EDD passes, waiting around for labour to start. You can avoid the worst of this void by planning some social activities such as going to the cinema or having supper with friends who won't mind if you have to cancel at the last moment. But don't succumb to invitations a long way from home without thinking through how you will get back to the hospital if your waters break. Above all, don't plan a drinks party at home to celebrate the birth because you may well be too exhausted to shine. Keep your diary blank as far as grand social occasions go.

Something to remember is that if you give a precise EDD to your family and friends, they will deluge you with phone calls on that day and each day after. For some reason this is incredibly irritating if your baby is late. If you have an answerphone, think about changing your message ('This is ..., thank you for calling, no, the baby hasn't arrived yet', etc.) so you don't end up continually apologising for not going into labour.

You will need to have a labour bag and a case ready-packed for your stay in hospital. Many pregnancy books suggest what should go in them. In case you haven't thought about this, we have provided lists at the back of the book. A superbly organised woman will put into the new baby car seat some suitable, loose-fitting (outsize!) day clothes for herself and a nightie and shawl for her new baby. Her husband just has to scoop this up as he leaves home to pick them up from hospital. This is a way of ensuring that the woman does not have to walk to the car in her nightie. He won't forget the baby clothes but he might forget yours.

7

Thinking ahead about your baby

This is more than daydreaming about how things will be; it means making a few decisions and plans, though not too many. One important principle is that you should be prepared to be flexible and consider your various options without committing yourself completely until your baby has been born. It is not necessary to be too ambitiously organised. Baby books can give a very daunting impression of life with a baby – they may have pages and pages on equipment and procedures.

There are a few things you simply must have in stock (nappies, vests and receiving or swaddling sheets – see page 215 about these) and it makes sense to get them beforehand, but you don't need to get absolutely everything. Some people approach childbirth with a siege mentality and overstock, rather like the behaviour you can see in a supermarket just before a Bank Holiday weekend. Although your opportunities for shopping will be curtailed in the first few weeks, life goes on after childbirth and you can still buy or borrow what you need when you need it. You cannot always predict what you may be given as presents, either. Although it is a good idea to lay in a large stash of food before the birth, the best policy for buying equipment and clothes is to get only the minimum beforehand.

THE LAYETTE (BABY GEAR AND EQUIPMENT)

Of course you will have started to get some baby gear together. Pregnancy books explain what this 'layette' consists of (we have included a list at the end of this book if you haven't got one). Keep one or two principles in mind:

- You probably don't need as much as you think.
- Keep all receipts in case you need to change things because your baby arrives bigger or smaller or a different sex than you imagined.
- A 9-pound baby is considerably larger than a 6-pound baby and will bypass the first size in vests and babygrows. (You may not know if you prefer babygrows or nighties until you actually have your baby.)
- Friends and relatives are often generous and give you bits and pieces so you can easily end up with duplicates.
- Everything has to be stored somewhere.

Incidentally, contrary to what used to be said, you don't actually need to wash everything before you use it. The exception are new towels which tend not to dry properly until they have been washed.

WHERE IS THE BABY GOING TO SLEEP?

There is no shortage of advice on this point, some of it forcefully expressed but without much in the way of solid fact or rationale to back it up. The short answer is that, by and large, he should sleep in whichever place you feel most comfortable about. Like many things in life about which you receive contradictory advice, it doesn't actually matter very much where he sleeps to begin with. It might be alongside your bed, at the foot of your bed, in a separate room or on the landing – anywhere that is convenient and within earshot or within reach of a baby-alarm. Consider the various options as they apply to your home but don't make a final decision until you come out of hospital. What seems proper or logical beforehand may not feel right to you later. In practice, most couples start off having their baby sleeping in a Moses basket with them in their bedroom.

Whether you should plan to have your baby in bed with you right from the start is an issue. Some ideologists advocate this but there are no emotional advantages for him and a few difficulties. There is a remote chance that he may overheat which is potentially dangerous. Your bed is unlikely to be big enough for three. That usually means that your husband moves out. Indeed, some women capitalise on this as the weeks wear on and use the baby in bed as a contraceptive.

If you have a big bed and it seems the right place yet you are worried that you or your husband will roll over on to him (which is very unlikely) you can wall off a space with a pillow, and also make sure that neither you nor your husband is drunk or out cold with a sleeping pill. On the other hand, if you are going to wall off a space with a pillow, your baby might as well be next to the bed. You can sense that we have just a few reservations about planning to have him *always* in bed with you though, of course, every parent takes their baby into their bed to sleep from time to time.

You may also find out later on that you are the type of mother who sleeps less well when your baby is in your bed. It is very common indeed for women to wake in the night in a confused panic as to whether their babies are or are not in the bed with them, and have or have not suffocated.

From the baby's point of view there is no one place that is psychologically more advantageous than any other. Apart from the minor reservation that we have about planning to have him in your bed as a permanent fixture, the only place where it is *wrong* for your baby to sleep is somewhere with which *you don't feel comfortable*.

DECISIONS ABOUT FEEDING

The decision to breast or bottle feed is like other aspects of babycare. You don't necessarily have to make a firm decision before you have your baby because you have time afterwards and what you eventually choose must feel right for both you and your baby. Some mothers will breast feed one of their children but not the other, not so much on account of their increasing experience but because the individual personalities of their babies mean that it feels right to give one a bottle, the other the breast.

One way of thinking about the decision is not to see it as a stark choice between breast and bottle but a question as to when you will transfer from breast to bottle. Before your milk comes through, the breast produces a yellowish fluid (colostrum) which is rich in protein, and especially antibodies against infection. There are therefore substantial advantages in putting your baby to the breast for the first few days to ensure he gets the goodies from the colostrum for which no substitute exists. You can transfer to the bottle from any time thereafter. Some women are sure they are not going to be able to face breast feeding but, having been encouraged, go on to find it perfectly all right. Our recommendation is to start by giving breast feeding a go and make up your mind later.

Breast milk has nutritional advantages over formula milk and has one or two other benefits such as providing better protection against infection and, possibly, against allergies too. It has, after all, more than a million years of development behind it. Once established, breast feeding is easier in the long term as there is absolutely no preparation involved. **All authorities agree it is the preferred method for most babies.**

If you are going to breast feed, assume everything is going to go well – it does for the vast majority of mothers. It is probably simpler than it is made out to be. One of the snags associated with breast feeding is that if it does prove tricky to establish, there are too many 'experts' with different advice. They usually have very definite views indeed so that you can easily get confused as a result. The truth is that there are very few breast feeding practices which apply to all mothers and all babies so that didactic, inflexible advice is inappropriate.

Although breast feeding is preferable, it is certainly not imperative and your baby will thrive perfectly well on a bottle. Formula milk is most definitely adequate for a baby to grow on. In the long term, it doesn't matter much which you opt for. You can't, for instance, tell which school-children were breast fed as babies. Bottle feeding enables your husband and others to help with feeds, especially at night and gives you more freedom during the day. It is also technically much easier to establish and therefore goes more smoothly in the early weeks.

If you do make up your mind that you are going to transfer very early from breast to bottle, buy the equipment before the birth. You then have time to practise all the rituals of cleaning, sterilising, formula preparation and warming before you have to do it for real in the presence of an urgently screaming, hungry baby.

Incidentally, you will need to buy some maternity bras – three if you are planning to breast feed and at least one even if you are planning to put your baby directly on to the bottle. It is important that you are fitted by someone who is specifically trained to fit nursing bras. She will know how much extra cup size to allow for when your milk comes through, as well as ensuring you have enough hooks to be able to tighten the bra when your rib cage returns to its original size. The ideal time to be fitted is when you are between 36 and 38 weeks' pregnant.

However you are going to feed, make sure you have a decent chair to sit in while you are doing so. This means an old-fashioned nursing chair if you can find one. Otherwise use a low-seated, high-backed, armless chair of the sort often found in bedrooms. You will probably need to buy extra pillows. You will need three to lean against when you are feeding in bed, the baby will lie on one placed on your lap (to bring him up to your breast) and you may need another pillow under your thighs to take your weight off painful episiotomy stitches.

NAMES

Unless you are quite sure of the sex of your future baby (and ultrasound is not completely reliable on this score, though amniocentesis is), be very careful not to get too hung up on the idea that you are going to have a baby of one particular sex. It is remarkably easy to become convinced you are going to have a girl, so that you choose only girls' names. You then get caught out badly when a boy arrives and each parent will panic that the other is secretly disappointed. Rehearse names of both sexes and, even then, wait to see what your new baby actually looks like before making a final decision.

Not all babies suit the name you have chosen and it rapidly becomes too late to change it. Don't enjoy a joke (which might take the form of an old family name) at your child's expense – if you have to include a totally unfashionable family name, put it second or third. Remember to consider the impact of infelicitous initials, shortenings and derived nicknames – you will probably know someone whose parents obviously didn't. Even if the two of you are able to agree on a shortlist of names, you will need to be prepared for the inevitable shock horror reactions of your family.

CIRCUMCISION

Bear in mind that most hospitals and most paediatricians nowadays are not in favour of routine circumcision, nor is it something which is usually available through the National Health Service, so if you want your baby boy circumcised you will need to make private arrangements (ask your general practitioner).

Think about it ahead of time and talk it over with your husband. Some circumcised fathers take it for granted that their son will be circumcised. Conversely, some wives of circumcised men assume wrongly that their husbands will automatically want a circumcised son. If you both view circumcision as a religious imperative then fine; if only one of you does, that's awkward and needs talking through. (For more details see Appendix 5 on page 225.)

8

Thinking ahead about your other (step-)children

Although this is a book for first-time mothers, some of these will already be step-mothers, perhaps with small children at home who will need to be thought about before their step-brother or step-sister is born.

You will obviously have told your child or children that they are going to have a new baby brother or sister. It is surprisingly common for women to worry unreasonably about the impact the new baby will have on an elder child's psyche – some women even worry that they will not have enough love to go round and include the baby they are carrying. You can start to act positively now to minimise difficulties later:

- Tell them what is going to happen; that you will go into hospital, who will look after them, that you will come back with the new baby, etc.
- Let them feel the bump and the baby's kicks if they want to.

- Allow older children to attend a late scan – if you have one. This enables them to 'see' the baby, which is an easy way of helping them confront the reality of the situation while there is time before its arrival to come to terms with it.
- Involve them as much as possible in the buying of baby equipment or clothes.
- Get them accustomed to the routine of a rest or quiet period in their room after lunch. This is *essential*.
- Get them used to spending time with their father and away from your side.
- Buy them a present that the new baby can give them – it must be something worthwhile, rather than a stocking present. It must also be wanted (this almost certainly means not educational)!

Problems with older children's jealousy of the new baby or their regression to immature behaviour are more likely to be a reaction to a change in *your* behaviour than the fact of the new baby's existence.

Although children can be understandably jealous of the way in which the new baby has taken pride of place in your affections, it has been shown that when a new baby enters the family, most mothers become sharper, more impatient and spend less time playing with their older children. The children sense this and resent it, not unreasonably. They may or may not take it out on the baby. It is often not so much jealousy of the baby as puzzled anger at the change in you and an inspired guess as to just who might be to blame for that.

If you know about the possibility that a new baby may change your attitude and behaviour like this, it should (in theory!) be easier for you to catch yourself doing it and balance things accordingly.

STAGE 2

In hospital

9

The first hour or so

So far we have been considering thinking ahead; planning for the baby well before he arrives. This is not a book about how a baby is born so we can skip the details of labour which are described in many other books and move to the moment of birth.

As your baby is being born you might hear a sucking noise. Because it is important that his nose is clear when he takes his first breath, the midwife will be clearing his nose and mouth with a small suction tube. When he takes his first breaths he may cry but some babies do not. In the old days, babies were hung upside down and slapped on the bottom to drain any fluid from their nose or mouth and shock them into breathing. This made all of them cry which reassured their parents but it is no longer thought to be a practice which is either civilised or necessary. Your baby may not cry but still be perfectly well.

Newborn babies look a bit blue and lifeless before they take their first breath. They do not turn pink until they have taken a few breaths, and even then the baby will probably look fairly blotchy for an hour or two, often with blue hands and feet.

At this stage your baby is still attached to the afterbirth (placenta) by the umbilical cord. The midwife will clamp this cord with plastic clips, then cut it. This does not hurt him or you. She may ask your husband if he would like to cut the cord and whether he takes her up on that is entirely up to him; he certainly shouldn't feel he has to.

Midwives sometimes suggest that your baby is laid on your tummy 'to help bonding'. This is a relatively new ritual for which there is no particular justification and, if you don't want this, say so. As far as getting close to your baby is concerned, it is better to hold him in your arms so that the two of you can look at each other but if you want to wait until the cord has stopped pulsating (and it doesn't matter if you do or don't) you will have to wait a minute or so until the cord is cut. This is because most cords aren't long enough to allow the mother to hold her baby comfortably whilst he is still attached. There is no urgency about any of this; so-called bonding is a matter of getting to know each other gradually. The first few minutes are not crucial for your longer-term relationship.

Very soon after your baby is born he will be taken to a resuscitation trolley, checked over quickly, weighed, measured and given an Apgar score. This is a routine assessment of the baby's general condition developed some 30 years ago. It will be repeated in another four minutes and involves the midwife or doctor examining him closely. He may be given a drop of vitamin K on his tongue or by injection to prevent haemorrhagic disease of the newborn, a rare but critical condition in which the baby's blood fails to clot so that he bleeds internally (and sometimes fatally) a few days or weeks after birth. Although different hospitals have different policies on vitamin K e is then wrapped in a blanket (because babies get cold quickly), name tags are put on his wrist and ankle and checked with yours before he is given back to you. Some hospitals use additional methods of identification. You may not want to hold your baby until he has been wrapped in a blanket. It doesn't matter what you do so long as *it feels right for you* at the time.

Immediately after your baby is born you may find yourself in tears of joy and relief but you are not abnormal if this does not happen. Quite commonly it is the father who is in tears and surprised at himself while the mother is saying 'Where's the tea?' If this happens, fathers are sometimes worried that the woman isn't 'bonding', but human feelings are much more complex than that. What it probably means is that she is exhausted and thirsty. It is interesting that the magic of birth not uncommonly affects fathers first and mothers a little later; while the men are coming down from their high, the mothers are warming up for theirs. Watching your baby being born is a remarkable privilege for fathers and can be a more powerful emotional experience than actually giving birth.

The first thought in your mind is likely to be 'Is my baby normal?' Nearly all (98 per cent) are, but you may not be prepared for what a normal newborn baby looks like:

- Wet.
- Maybe a bluish colour.
- Perhaps a little blood on him – this will be your blood rather than his.
- Sometimes a bit slippery because of a covering of a creamy substance called vernix.
- Rather loose reddish skin.
- Asymmetrically shaped head – sometimes alarmingly so.
- Often a puffy face.
- Huge scrotum or large labia and sometimes breast

development (all as a result of the temporary effect of your hormones which have crossed the placenta).
- Sometimes fine hair on temples, forehead, shoulders and back.
- Sometimes small red 'stork's beak' marks on the back of the neck, on the nose or eyelids.
- The 'wrong' coloured hair (blond children are often born with dark hair).

Over the next few days and weeks, all these unexpected features will fade. Difficult or protracted deliveries leave their own marks which will also disappear. The skull bones are free to move as the baby progresses through the mother's pelvis so the baby's head may seem uneven. Forceps can leave temporary bruising marks on the cheeks and a ventouse (suction) delivery often leaves a ring mark with some swelling on the scalp. There may be a small mark on his head if a blood sample has been taken from it during labour or a monitor clip has been attached. All these marks will vanish completely.

This might sound as though you would feel squeamish about your new baby (and many pregnant women secretly worry about just this) but they are actually cuddly, very appealing and smell nice. New babies are good news.

Your midwife may encourage you to put your baby to the breast because this will help your uterus to contract down. Even if you have decided to bottle feed from the start, this is a good idea (if you can face it and are not too exhausted). Although it is assumed that this is a natural activity, it is common to feel self-conscious the first time you put your baby to the breast. You may find it difficult to hold the baby and find a comfortable position if you have a drip in your arm. You may also feel nervous about holding him safely and generally getting things right.

THE FIRST HOUR OR SO

Fathers need to recognise that it often feels a bit awkward when neither of you have done it before and realise that mothers, however experienced they may be with other people's babies, are likely to feel vulnerable, self-conscious and lacking in self-confidence when it comes to their own first baby. Be prepared for the fact that not all babies suckle immediately.

A few minutes after the baby is born the placenta is delivered and taken away. It has done its job and you and your baby no longer need it. It slips away from you painlessly but somewhat messily, looking like a large lump of raw liver. Before it is delivered there will have been virtually no blood or anything that may make fathers feel squeamish, but at this stage fathers who do not like the sight of blood should stay at the head end of the bed. The same applies if you need any stitching up afterwards.

We are not very sold on the idea of eating your own placenta. There was a short-lived fad for this some years ago based on the observation that a number of mammals do so in order to avoid detection by predators and to conserve nutrition. Neither reason seems relevant today.

If you have had an episiotomy or a tear you will need stitches. These are put in by a midwife or doctor using a local anaesthetic or by topping up the epidural if you had one. While this is being done, your feet may be put up in stirrups (slings attached to upright poles at the end of the bed) so that the stitcher can see what she or he is doing. The stitching should not be painful and if it is say so! No one wants you to suffer and the stitcher can adjust the local anaesthetic. Alternatively you can keep going with the gas and air. Fathers should take responsibility for checking that you are pain-free as many women feel that, having coped with childbirth, they ought to be able to manage the lesser pain of stitching and don't want to cause a fuss by complaining. Nevertheless, insufficient pain relief can result in a traumatic memory which can and should always be avoided.

Once the stitches are in, it is a good idea to attempt five short, quick pelvic floor lifts while the anaesthetic is still working. This won't burst the stitches, in fact it will bring the stitch line together (if you manage to get any movement at all). It will start the pelvic floor muscle nerve pathways working again after delivery, and it will stimulate blood flow to the area which speeds up healing.

Once the delivery activities are over you will be helped to wash and change into a clean nightie and given a sanitary towel since you will continue to lose quite a lot of blood-stained fluid (lochia) from where the placenta was attached to your uterus. The amount of this bleeding can be surprising – it is prudent not to put on your best nightie. You will be given a cup of tea and something to eat (probably not as much as you would like, so tuck into anything you have brought with you).

Your baby is likely to be quiet now – he may even fall asleep – and you will have an hour or so to rest together. Make the most of this. It is usually a magical time for you both as a couple. The important thing is that you now have your baby. However, it is only fair to say that it is not uncommon for some women to experience violent shivering or to be sick directly after birth which obviously means the magic bit will have to wait until later.

Take some photographs – you will regret it if you don't. Polaroids can be shown to visitors but you don't get such a good picture to keep.

Only when you are settled should the father leave you and make the necessary phone calls. Correct protocol is for him to phone your mother before his – it is important that he gets this right!

10

The 'bonding' business

During the 1970s, a number of healthcare professionals became convinced that the first few days of a baby's life were crucial in establishing an emotional bond between mother and child and the healthy development of the child. Two theories combined to produce this idea.

Firstly, early studies of premature babies who had been separated from their mothers soon after birth and placed in incubators because they had breathing troubles suggested that some of the mothers of these children had trouble loving their babies. Secondly, the view of Leboyer, a French obstetrician, that childbirth was a violent transition from a kindly intrauterine environment to a harsh external world, led him to advocate ways in which birth could be made less traumatic for the baby.

Both these aspects were combined with a widely held assumption (now questioned) that a child's development is shaped more by early life circumstances than by later ones.

The early studies on premature babies and their separation from their mothers led to some theorising and some further scientific study. The theory which emerged stated that the first few days of a baby's life were a sensitive period in which the mother formed an emotional bond with her baby. For this to happen, she had to have skin-to-skin contact with him for several hours a day. If this was prevented by separation, then it was held that there was a risk that she would never achieve truly loving feelings towards him, there would be a failure of maternal 'bonding' and an increased likelihood of future child abuse. It was also thought that the baby's development would be slowed in some areas.

When this was combined with Leboyer's suggestions, the practice of placing a newborn baby on to the mother's belly 'to help the bonding' arose and this has led to a number of mothers becoming apprehensive about not bonding with their babies. The views of Leboyer are just that – opinions without any scientific evidence to support them. The scientific findings relevant to the separation issue have changed over the years as the studies exploring the area have become more sophisticated and a number of earlier complications ironed out. What emerges from the more recent work is a very different picture from the earlier theory.

The current view is that:

- Separation of mother and new baby does not affect most mothers' abilities to bond to their babies at all.
- Occasionally, a new mother does find it hard to experience spontaneous feelings of love and warmth towards her baby. There are a number of reasons for this: she may be exhausted; she may be frightened that her baby will die (especially if he has to be put into an incubator) and so she withholds her feelings; the baby might be premature or malformed and not look like the baby she was expecting; or she may lack self-

confidence and feel that she will not be able to care for the baby.
- This doesn't usually matter. New mothers who have not felt immediate feelings of love for their babies discover these feelings within a few days or weeks in nearly all cases. The microscopic number for whom this doesn't happen have continuing severe life stresses (such as homelessness or being abandoned by their husband) which drain and divert them emotionally. What counts in such instances is what is going on at the time, not what happened in the first few days of their baby's life.
- It often takes time to fall in love with your baby. Human relationships are not so mechanical that they can be switched on and off by a single event.
- As far as the child's later development is concerned, there are no apparent long-term consequences of so-called bonding failure in the first few days of life.

Delivering the baby on to your tummy for the sole purpose of promoting 'bonding' is a nonsense. Allowing a mother and baby to get to know each other fact-to-face after birth is much more to the point. If a baby is held in his mother's arms, her face is just the right distance away from him to bring it into focus for his eyes. Newborn babies are usually alert, actively looking around and particularly responsive to their mother's voice and face. Very bright lights will cause a baby to screw up his eyes so a sensitive hospital will dim the lights accordingly. Wanting to pick your baby up and hold him in your arms is a natural thing to do. If you want your baby on your tummy, all well and good. But don't imagine that it will seal an emotional contract between the two of you.

The whole idea of early 'bonding' has become confused

with a different process which first starts much later at about six months when the baby begins to cling to a particular person, usually his mother, and cries if she leaves him. This develops into a close emotional relationship over a period of months and certainly is a powerful influence on the baby's emotional development. Confusingly, this very different process, which has nothing to do with the mother's feelings just after birth, is sometimes called 'affectional bonding', though 'attachment' is a more usual term. It has more to do with the baby's emotions than the mother's.

Although recent findings have largely dispelled the earlier assumption that bonding is a crucial, once-and-for-all, superglue-like process, the whole business has done much to humanise the care of mothers and new babies. Nowadays, nobody believes (as they once did) that all new babies are best nursed in incubators away from their mothers, and no mother should experience her baby being removed from her without good reason. One perfectly good reason is when she asks for a break.

The message for mothers is simple. Don't panic. You may or may not fall in love with your baby immediately. It doesn't matter. If you are worried that you will not, then the paradox is that you are the sort of person who will become a caring, loving parent. The right thing to do nearly always turns out to be what seems right for you and your baby at the time. You need not feel that you have to go along with someone else's ideas about the proper thing to do if it feels wrong. For instance, you are quite entitled to ask for your baby to be taken away so that you can get some sleep; don't feel guilty or apprehensive that you will disturb some magical process.

11

Getting it right and the myth of the perfect start

Many first-time mothers are determined to get it right, absolutely from the beginning. They want to give their baby the perfect start and plan accordingly. However, this can go awry: minor complications may mean the carefully constructed birth plan has to go out of the window so that the mother feels she has failed irrevocably.

Things may, indeed, not turn out as you intended. Your baby and your body may have different ideas from you as to how the birth will progress. There is not much you can do about your labour if your baby has not manoeuvred himself into a head-down position or if your pelvis proves to be too small for the delivery. As far as labour is concerned, you just can't plan everything on your own and it is not likely to be the fault of the obstetrician or midwife if you can't have the 'natural' birth you wanted. *It certainly won't be your fault either*. Approach childbirth with realistic expectations and an open mind and continue to keep your mind open when it comes to looking after your new baby.

Babies are remarkably parent-proof. They are also tough enough to weather all sorts of mishaps like early or difficult births, most infections or feeding problems. Nature does not depend upon things going perfectly and budgets for minor complications.

Nor are early life circumstances as overwhelmingly important for your baby's future personality as most people think. It is a common fallacy to think that the earlier an influence on a child, the more powerful it will be. If you were firing an arrow at a target, a small difference in your aim would mean a huge difference in where the arrow eventually ended up. The temptation is to think that children are like this – give them an ideal start and they will develop ideally; get it slightly wrong at the start and disaster will follow later in life. But the development of children and young adults is just not like that. It depends on processes rather than events.

Thus, for the vast majority of aspects of development, it is *continuing* influences that have the most powerful effects. Early influences can become important when they continue (and therefore act for a longer time than influences which arise later in life), not just because they are early. In other words an early event in itself is not likely to be important unless it persists and turns from an event into a constant process. Missing a meal is not important but continually being starved would be.

Obviously, we have to exclude devastating physical illnesses or injuries from this, but many less serious physical problems which seem alarming at the time can have their effects diluted by good-enough care over the childhood years. Even babies who appear to have suffered brain injury during birth can catch up on their development provided they experience adequate parenting subsequently.

In one study, the effect of serious birth complications was to slow babies' developmental progress and this could be shown by assessing them at one year of age. But in good-quality homes these babies had caught up with normal developmental expectations by the time they were ten years old and were then indistinguishable from babies who had entirely normal births. Sadly, in very poor-quality homes with poverty, parental strife and some neglect, the development of babies with serious birth complications was not only slow at one year but became worse with time and they fell even further behind. What seems to matter is what goes on over time. So, do not be seduced by the myth of the perfect start. It may be a nice thing to aim for but it is not likely to be your fault if you cannot achieve it and it is certainly not crucial for your baby.

Every mother remembers something dreadful which she allowed to happen to her baby – letting him fall out of his basket or realising too late that he had been crying with hunger for hours. Sometimes there is a haunting fear that the baby will remember the incident all his life, holding it as an accusation against his mother for not being a perfect parent. Actually, it is virtually unknown for anyone to remember experiences from their first two years of life. Even after that, memories are extremely fragmentary. Most people have grave difficulty remembering anything much before the age of three.

Quite a lot of thinking assumes that babies are passive and therefore it is up to their parents to get everything right for them. But, as we have pointed out earlier, babies take an active part in their development. They stimulate you into doing things for them. They elicit feelings, attitudes and actions from you. Right from the start they establish a relationship with you and their development progresses within a setting of human relationships. They are not like plants which require merely that you provide water, light and potting compost for their growth. Children mature in a matrix of relationships within which they are not passive but active contributors. In a way this never stops because personal, as opposed to physical, development never stops. It means that there continue to be opportunities for things to go right and correct themselves, even if they appear to have gone wrong. Hang on to the idea that, in development, nothing is for ever.

12

The postnatal ward

After your baby has been born and you have been tidied up you will be moved to a bed in a hospital postnatal ward. Your baby will be in a cot beside you and probably lying quietly. You can, in theory, sleep. In practice, you probably won't as you will still be on a high following the birth, or panicking about what you're supposed to do if your baby cries. If you are lucky enough to doze off you will be woken promptly by the crying of somebody else's baby or the arrival in the ward of another recently delivered mother as her trolley collides with the metal plate on the ward doors. Be prepared to spend much of the first night (and subsequent nights) awake. In the old days you would have been given a sleeping pill and the baby taken away for the night; probably a good idea but currently unfashionable.

If you have had an epidural, it may have weakened the control over your leg muscles. Don't go to the loo on your own until you have been told that it is safe, otherwise you may find your knees giving way before you get there. Ring the buzzer by your bed for a nurse to go with you.

YOUR PELVIC FLOOR

This is likely to feel rather sore. How sore will obviously depend on how easily your baby was delivered. Some women will have an intact (though stretched) pelvic floor, but most will have stitches. The number of stitches you may have varies enormously, depending on the size and position of your baby during delivery. At one end of the spectrum you may have a couple of stitches following a small tear and at the other extreme it might seem that your entire pelvic floor is stitched up.

Most forceps deliveries necessitate an episiotomy (a small cut to widen the vaginal opening further) and different types of forceps require different sized cuts and therefore different numbers of stitches. Kielland's forceps, which have to be used in order to rotate a baby's head, tend to leave women feeling rather more sore and bruised than simple 'lift out' forceps such as Wrigley's. If the woman in the next bed to you claims that she had forceps yet is leaping around with alarming agility while you can't sit down, don't panic that something has gone wrong; it's just that she probably had the smaller version.

You may also have developed a thrombosed external pile (peri-anal haematoma) which is a burst blood vessel under the skin around the anus. This can be appallingly painful but is self-limiting. Most will clear up within ten days without needing any treatment, but meanwhile it may help to lie on the bed with your bottom on a pillow for as much of your time as possible.

If your labour was long and you had a difficult second stage, you might find you have aching or sore muscles. You may even discover that you have bloodshot eyes (especially if you missed the antenatal class that concentrated on 'pushing' effectively).

HOW BEST TO HELP YOUR RECOVERY

Do not panic. Your stitches will heal, the muscles will return to normal – or even better than before.

When offered pain relief, take it if you need it. It does go into the breast milk but it doesn't matter. No hospital is going to give you medicines that will harm your baby.

Continue your pelvic floor exercises in groups of five, ten times a day (a total of at least 50 a day) however sore your stitches are and even if you have got painful external piles. The muscles will feel rather spongy at first. The exercises actually help the healing process by increasing the blood supply to the area and dispersing the swelling. Any increase in intra-abdominal pressure will put a strain on your episiotomy stitches and already stretched muscles, so try to remember to tighten your pelvic floor muscles whenever you cough, laugh, sneeze or get up from sitting. Obstetric physiotherapists are trained to help with crutch and bottom problems – ask to see one if you are in a lot of pain.

Wash your bottom twice daily in a bidet if there is one. Pat the area dry with a paper towel and finish drying the stitches with a hair-dryer, obviously ensuring the hair-dryer does not get too hot. (This is best tackled behind your curtains when you are not expecting visitors!) Finish off with five pelvic floor exercises, as usual.

At some stage (usually about 24 hours after delivery) you are going to have to face the daunting task of opening your bowels. (Some people call this the fourth stage of labour!) Most women become fairly constipated in hospital after having had a baby, which doesn't make things any easier. This is partly because they get dehydrated during labour, partly because of a change in routine and diet. Rather than relying on what is often low-fibre hospital food, it may help to take in your own supply of what you normally have for breakfast with extra high-fibre cereal, dried fruit or whatever helps to keep your bowels ticking over.

If you have stitches, you are also likely to be worrying that you will be unable to open your bowels without the world falling out of your bottom. When attempting to defaecate, it will be much better for your pelvic floor and easier for you if you give the stitch line counter-pressure while you are bearing down. Take a fresh sanitary pad into the loo with you, fold it in two and, with one hand, hold the folded pad firmly against the stitch line to give counter-pressure as you relax your pelvic floor and gently try to defaecate. (It is usually at this point that there is a bang on the loo door and a voice tells you accusingly that your baby is crying.) If you have had a Caesarean section the same principle applies but you apply counter-pressure to your abdominal scar.

LOCHIA

For the first few days you will bleed quite heavily from your vagina in the same way as you would if you were having a very heavy period, but rather more so. Bloody fluid seeps from the site where the placenta was attached to the wall of the uterus. This is painless and quite normal. The midwives may seem unreasonably curious as to its colour and smell but this is because they want to check that all is progressing normally with no infection or bits of placenta ('retained products') left behind. There shouldn't be any large clots; if there are, save them on your sanitary towel if possible and show them to the midwife.

PICKING UP YOUR BABY

Don't be inhibited about picking up your baby when you feel like it. Cradle his head with your fingers as you do so. He needs to be handled and to get to know you. After a few days he can recognise your face, voice and smell and will respond to you more than any other person. Your face is his first plaything and in a few weeks' time you will see his smile when he sees you and you talk to him. Start on it now: pick him up and talk to him in a light tone using any silly phrase which comes to mind. Sing to him softly and tell him what you think of him or what is going on. It doesn't really matter what you say but a repetitive, high-pitched, sing-song voice appeals. Get him used to the sound of you. Pull faces at him so that he learns all the appearances of your face. Kiss and cuddle him, you won't break anything. Nor will you 'spoil' him by picking him up. Some things about your baby might alarm you:

- His umbilical stump and its clip may look distinctly off-putting and about to snap off dangerously. It won't, it will separate gradually, usually dropping off within the first ten days. The midwives will show you how to clean it. Most mothers fold the top of the nappy below it so that urine doesn't seep into the umbilical area. It is not a disaster if it does and you don't have to have nappies with a cut-out for the umbilical stump.
- Newborn babies have little control over their heads which roll around alarmingly and need supporting by your fingers as you pick them up.
- Although you probably knew that a baby has two soft patches (fontanelles) in his skull, it is a bit of a jolt when you feel them for the first time. There is a membrane under the skin which is much tougher than

you think and you won't puncture it by accident.
- A scalp monitor may leave a small scab of dried blood on the top of your baby's head, and forceps can produce bruise marks or scratches on his face. These will disappear completely.
- Many newborn babies appear to have a squint. This becomes less evident as they learn to coordinate their eye movements.
- Their first bowel movement is greenish-black and sticky, this being the meconium which fills the bowels of babies in the womb.
- Some babies develop a mild jaundice for a few days after their birth because their livers are not yet working to full capacity. This might need some ultra-violet light therapy to disperse it but is otherwise not a problem, except that affected babies are often rather drowsy and suckle weakly. They therefore may need to be woken up for feeds (perhaps every three hours during the day and every four hours at night once your milk is through).

VISITORS

These need to be monitored by your husband. We carried out a survey in which we asked new mothers about their experiences in hospital. They said that the most helpful contribution their husbands made was shielding them from too many visitors. Your husband must make sure that, when he tells people about your new baby, he finds out when they plan to visit you.

People in hospital are trapped and cannot escape the visitor who stays too long. A newly delivered mother will not enjoy the necessary courtesies of introducing elderly relatives to current mates (and sustaining the conversation), when all she really wants to do is disappear into the lavatory before tackling another feed. Nor is she going to find it easy to attempt to breast feed in front of a well-meaning male work colleague or her father-in-law – however uninhibited she may be under normal circumstances. Husbands can try to ensure that she is not exposed to any 'surprise' visits.

Your husband has to ensure that you and he have enough time on your own together with your baby. He is your most important visitor and there must be time for the two of you to see each other alone. As he will probably still be at work, this is most likely to be in the evening. During this time he can look after the baby while you have a bath or grab an ST and head for the loo for another session with your stitch line, safe from the worry that your baby will need attention. You can also discuss together such matters as names, announcements, the christening, and what to do about particular visitors. He will need to wash and iron any dirty clothes you give him, returning these as quickly as possible, and go shopping on your behalf for fruit, food and equipment as necessary.

What quite often follows from this is that only the afternoons are available for other visitors. This has its own rationing effect. While you are in hospital the only other visitors who are really important are your parents and his; other people can visit you when you return home. It is probably wise for your husband to tell visitors that fifteen minutes is enough. If you have other children, less than this is enough. Pre-school children are not only exhausting but remarkably adept at preventing or interrupting conversations between their parents. They just need to check that you are all right and that there really is a baby. This doesn't take long and they become tiring if they stay longer. Give them a good hug and tell them when you'll be home.

If people bring presents for the baby, keep a record so that you can scribble a thank-you note later. Try to get your correspondence (birth announcement cards and thank-you notes) done while you are in hospital – there will be even less time once you get home. It is your husband's job to place the birth announcement in the newspaper.

STARTING TO BREAST FEED YOUR BABY

Your milk won't begin to come through until three to four days after delivery. You do, however, need to put your baby to the breast before then. Start as soon as you feel up to it. Before they start churning out milk, the breasts produce a small amount of a cloudy fluid called colostrum. This contains antibodies against infection as well as other goodies and is, from the baby's point of view, well worth having. The suckling of your baby will also help stimulate the release of hormones which kick-start the lactation process (though if for any reason you can't put your baby to the breast, the milk will still come through eventually).

Your first try at breast feeding must be supervised by the sister or a senior midwife if at all possible. It is often a good idea to try to enlist the help of the midwife who delivered you – you know and trust her, and she will be particularly keen to help you over this first hurdle. She will ensure your baby is latching on properly, taking both the nipple and the areola (brown area around it) into his mouth rather than hanging on to the nipple only, which will make it sore. She will check you are releasing his suction vacuum correctly by putting your finger into his mouth (not by pinching his nose or pulling him away).

Babies don't need milk for the first three days. They are

designed to go without, being born with a good reserve supply of nutrition. It is quite usual for them to lose up to 10 per cent of their birth weight in the first five days. Babies vary enormously, one from another, during these early days. Some are very sleepy and seem to be quite uninterested in feeding whilst others are keen to suckle immediately and seem to be starving. Unfortunately, you are likely to worry on both accounts.

If your baby is disinterested in feeding you may be told (or threatened!) that your milk won't come in unless he suckles all the time. It will – in some cultures the baby is never put to the breast until the mother begins to lactate. You are also likely to worry if he wants to suckle all the time in case you are starving him. Normally, babies do not need bottles of formula milk in the first three days, though you may be offered these (especially at night!). You don't have to be browbeaten into giving a bottle of milk by someone saying that your baby is hungry, unless this is on the advice of a paediatrician. The risk is that your baby becomes overfed and won't suckle.

There are two exceptions to all this. Babies who have not grown adequately during pregnancy are sometimes unable to regulate their own blood sugar level well enough and need early feeding. Very heavy babies sometimes can't settle at all because they are genuinely starving hungry. Your paediatrician will tell you if this is the case.

During the first three days you and your baby start to get into the swing of things as far as feeding is concerned. This is a 'running-in period' before the real thing, so don't leave your baby suckling for a long period without making sure that he is latching on correctly with the whole of the brown areola (area around the nipple) in his mouth. If he sucks vigorously with a poor attachment you will get sore nipples before you have even started to lactate.

PRIMARY ENGORGEMENT

You will know when your milk comes through because your breasts will swell as the new milk distends them. In a few women, this is so dramatic that their breasts become distended up to three bra cup sizes so that they are enormous, tender, or sometimes extremely painful (it may feel as though they have been hit with a cricket bat). This is known as primary engorgement. The breasts can also become so rounded that there is not enough areola and nipple for a baby to latch on to properly. Should this happen to you, do not despair. It is a temporary phase and will pass within 48 hours. While it lasts it can be pretty unpleasant and you can get the feeling that you don't know where to put yourself. Your breasts must be well supported and you will be grateful that you had the foresight to buy a well-fitting maternity bra, even though you thought it looked ghastly as the time. Properly supported, your breasts will feel more comfortable (and less likely to develop stretch marks). It often helps to rest cold flannels on your breasts after a feed. Let them stay there for a good fifteen minutes and when you put your bra back on, tuck a fresh cabbage leaf into each bra cup. Although *warm* flannels on your breasts or a bath before a feed can help your milk flow, *avoid hot* flannels as these dilate your blood vessels and can make engorgement worse. In any case, tell the ward sister; she may apply a breast pump if things become desperate. This is not applied routinely as it can encourage the breast to produce even more milk. You may also need to take some painkillers such as paracetamol.

CONTINUING TO TRY TO BREAST FEED YOUR BABY

The whole topic of breast feeding generates a staggering amount of contradictory advice from all quarters, professional and lay. Everyone is an expert! In fact, all professionals have the same objectives in mind – your baby should receive some colostrum in the first three days, sucking enough to keep him settled and content, while lactation gets under way as soon and as easily as possible. Thereafter he should have enough milk to put on about an ounce a day so he regains his birth weight somewhere between the tenth and fourteenth day (or even before). It is in the details of feeding practice that advice varies and can be confusing. Don't panic, the details aren't important.

One breast or two?

Some midwives argue for the baby to be fed from only one breast per feed 'so that he gets his pudding' or hind-milk – the thicker milk from the back of the breast which is especially rich in fat. They will also have been taught that it is important for each breast to be *completely* emptied at each feed – which is more likely to happen if the baby is only offered the one. Other midwives will suggest swigs from alternate breasts to 'balance' both breasts (which might be kinder to your appearance), and is what several millions of mothers and babies have been doing up to now. If pushed, we would argue for the latter approach, since it seems to be rooted in common sense, but the main point is that it doesn't really matter. A recent study has shown how adept babies are at regulating their own intake of fat. (If you decide to opt for two breasts per feed, put a safety pin in the bra strap of the second breast to remind you to start with that one next feed time.) Other topics upon which you will hear differing advice are how often to feed and how long to feed.

How often?

How frequently you feed your baby is largely up to him – as a rough rule of thumb, most new babies will want to suckle about every two to three hours during the day. Small babies will demand relatively more frequent feeds than heavier babies. At night, a longer interval between feeds is perfectly all right (unless he is jaundiced: see above) and four hours or a little longer is quite reasonable. In fact, if you are lucky enough to have a baby who sleeps for a long period during the night, there is no need to wake him for a feed before six hours. Most newborn babies will want between six and ten feeds during a 24-hour period, but don't even think about routines at this stage.

How long?

In these first few days, the length of a feed is a question which is bound up with the potential problem of sore nipples. Sore or cracked nipples are horribly painful and, from our experience, the commonest reason for women to decide that breast feeding is not for them. They occur as a result of the baby not being latched on properly and from too much suckling too soon. Fair-skinned mothers are particularly vulnerable as are those that burn easily in the sun; both being signs of a delicate skin.

When the midwife or feeding sister has helped you put your baby on to the breast correctly, she is likely to suggest how long your baby should be allowed to feed. Some midwives will suggest you feed him for a short period of time – a few minutes – and some will tell you to keep him plugged on for as long as possible. Current trends are in favour of the latter approach. Much will depend on your baby (see above) as quite a few seem to be totally disinterested and have to be coaxed to suckle at all. On the other hand, some babies have a very powerful suck immediately and, if left suckling too long, can readily produce sore nipples unless properly latched on.

Because there are all of these considerations – proper latching on, strength of suck and type of skin – no simple rule applies. The vast majority of mothers find that it helps to gradually build up the length of time that the baby is allowed to suckle in the first days before the milk comes through. This gives nipples which, under normal circumstances, aren't used to being vigorously sucked every two hours a little time to get used to the new activity that is going on, and adapt accordingly. Unfamiliar use produces soreness. (If on the first day of spring you did a whole day's vigorous digging in the garden, your hands would be very sore indeed.) So it seems more sensible to let your baby feed for short periods initially, building up to around ten to fifteen minutes on each breast (or 20 to 30 minutes on one breast) by day four.

Sitting in a comfortable position to feed

Some hospitals do not like you feeding the baby in bed and prefer you to be in a chair. Wherever you feed, if you have a crutch full of bruises or stitches, sitting while feeding will be very uncomfortable but it is important for you to take the trouble to make yourself as comfortable as you possibly can. Any discomfort or pain you may be experiencing will certainly not facilitate your milk flow, and you may be sitting for half-an-hour or so. If you can find a comfortable position it will help you settle into feeding. Some wards

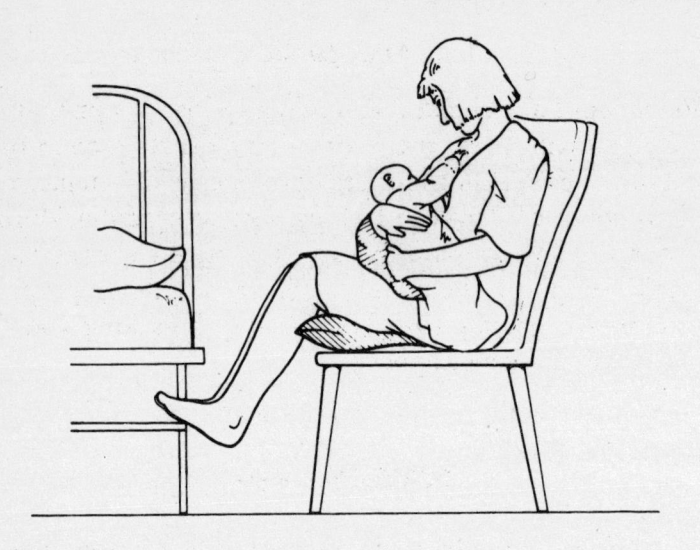

Figure 8 Sitting with pillows under thighs

provide a rubber ring to sit on. Actually a pillow doubled over along its long axis (the opposite to how you would instinctively fold a pillow) and put under your thighs as close to your buttocks as possible is just as effective. Both devices take your body weight off the stitches.

You should sit well back in the chair and support your feet if necessary (perhaps on the bar underneath your hospital bed). You can take the strain off your back and shoulders by supporting the baby on another pillow across your lap so that you are bringing baby to breast rather than breast to baby. Once he is latched on comfortably, drop your shoulders and close your eyes to rest for a few minutes.

After-pains

When your baby suckles, you may experience some 'after-pains' though these are more common in second-time mothers. The suckling releases hormones which make your uterus contract. This can feel just like contractions during labour and be very painful, especially with a second baby, but they do mean the uterus is contracting down properly to its pre-pregnancy size. Try the deep breathing you did during labour if this happens.

BOTTLE FEEDING

Try to feed your baby with your colostrum if you can; he will benefit from it. If not, most hospitals will suggest you start your baby on formula milk, often on the first day and show you how to feed him. Your breasts will still fill with milk. It is not current practice to give you any medication to 'dry the milk up' as this doesn't actually work very well. Wear a well-fitting bra with the straps tightened and ask for paracetamol if your breasts are very painful (see 'Primary Engorgement' above). It will take a few days for your breasts to get the message that they are not being required to produce milk and it will then be slowly reabsorbed. As when breast feeding, once your baby is happily guzzling, use this time to drop your shoulders and relax.

YOUR FIRST BATH

Feeling very sweaty while in hospital after having a baby is common, especially if you put on a lot of weight whilst pregnant. You will look forward to having a bath but might experience a sinking heart the first time that you strip off and have a chance to look at youself in private. The bulge will not yet have gone and you will look at least three (often six) months' pregnant. The skin on your tummy will look like orange peel or rumpled crêpe paper. So it does on other women's too; it will go. If you have had a Caesarean section there will be an alarming wad of flab which forms a 'shelf' above the incision. This, too, subsides with time. The linea nigra or pigmented line running up the middle is sometimes even more evident after you have had your baby than before, as are bright purple stretch marks on your lower tummy. All these will gradually fade over the next few months.

POSTNATAL EXERCISES

You should be seen by a physiotherapist while you are in hospital. With any luck she will be an obstetric physiotherapist, a specialist with postgraduate training. She will make sure you know how to carry out proper pelvic floor exercises and will introduce you to some basic routines which you can carry out on your bed to get your tummy muscles back into shape. This is not just cosmetic; these muscles are crucial in preventing low back strain. She may well leave you a sheet explaining future exercises (if not, we have included one at the back of this book). You will probably be keen to follow her tummy muscle exercises but what is *more important* is getting into the habit of holding your tummy in when standing or walking. This gets the tone back into the muscles, protecting your back and correcting your posture as you return to your pre-pregnant state. It is important to get good muscle tone *before* starting real strengthening exercises.

Remember that obstetric physiotherapists are also trained to help you with crutch and bottom problems if you have any.

BABY BLUES/MATERNITY BLUES/THREE-DAY BLUES

On about the third day after birth, more or less at the time that your milk comes through, you may, like many women, find yourself in tears for trivial reasons. At the same time you experience a heightened sensitivity to criticism or problems facing you. Your husband may seem unable to do anything right or the casual comments of visitors sound to you like damning indictments. If your first attempts at breast feeding are less than successful, you are likely to feel a complete failure. Your baby may need phototherapy (going under the lights) for jaundice and it feels like the end of the world. You take everything personally, have difficulty concentrating and may well feel irritable, anxious or panicky as to whether you will be able to cope with your baby. ('Why on earth didn't we book a maternity nurse?') This feels confusing and you may find yourself apologising for weeping.

It *isn't* postnatal depression, in fact it isn't really depression at all but a short-lived state of emotional turmoil which is at its height on the fifth day after birth. Some women are not affected (and therefore neither are their husbands). The simplest explanation is that it is an emotional upheaval connected with a peak in the hormonal changes following childbirth. It passes after a day or two and needs no medical treatment, but it is helpful for you both to understand that it is perfectly normal.

Unfortunately it is increasingly common for National Health Service hospitals to send new mothers home on the third day so that they can increase the use of hospital beds. From the mother's point of view it is probably the worst day they could choose.

SOME OTHER PEOPLE

If you are on a ward with someone who has had a Caesarean section, one of the most helpful things you can do for her is offer to lift her baby in and out of the cot for the first few days as she will find lifting painful, perhaps to the point where it is impossible.

If a woman's baby is seriously ill in the special care baby unit, don't ignore her – it helps enormously if you ask how her baby is and are able to commiserate appropriately. The same is even more true if her baby dies; the worst you can do is ignore her.

At some stage before you go home, an alarmingly young paediatrician will come to check over your baby as a matter of routine. Don't be afraid to ask questions during the examination (though not while he or she is listening to the heart).

Just when your crutch is at its most painful, the family planning sister comes round and starts talking about sex. Hear her out – she is an expert and you may well learn something. For instance, it is possible to conceive in the first six weeks after childbirth (believe it or not, it is also possible, albeit not usual, to have sex in the first six weeks after childbirth).

You might also have a visit from the chaplain who is, *par excellence*, a sympathetic ear (which you might welcome).

STAGE 3

At home

13

Coming home: the first few days

This section takes you up to roughly the end of your baby's first week. Most first-time mothers are better off staying in hospital for five days (even if the maternity nurse is already booked and waiting at home) though unfortunately it is fashionable for hospitals to discharge women on the third day. Second- or third-time mothers are more confident and will usually opt to come home after 48 hours. Mothers who have had a Caesarean section will need to stay in hospital for about six days, regardless of whether it is their first or a subsequent baby.

Given the choice, don't come home on the third or fourth day. This is when your milk is coming in, your breasts might be painfully engorged, and an acute attack of the baby blues is a real possibility. Enough is enough.

Coming home is the time when a husband comes in particularly handy. (If you haven't got one or he can't prise himself away from his job, recruit a friend.) He should clear his day, turn up at the hospital on time with a car parked as close to the entrance as possible, and be prepared to wait. If necessary, he brings your day clothes (not your tight jeans) and a shawl and clean clothes for the baby. Those women who have planned ahead will have packed suitable clothes for themselves and their baby in a child's car seat so that their husbands can just scoop this up on their way out of the house.

You may be secretly nervous about the drive home, given your husband's tendency to sublimate his sexual frustration into challenging roadmanship. As it happens, it is remarkable how new parenthood calms the most vigorous male driver but there is a genuine issue about the safety of babies in cars. The law in Britain states that the baby must go in a child's car seat which is a nightmare if you've never fiddled with a child seat before. In theory, you are no longer allowed to travel home sitting in the back of the car holding your baby. There is thus the possibility that you, the nurse and your husband will all stand in the rain while everyone tries to work out or tell each other how to get a tiny baby into a new car seat. All this is best avoided by taking the car seat up to the ward and putting your baby into it there. Here you have time to adjust the shoulder straps so that they fit and to work out how to fit the crutch strap between the legs of a swaddled baby.

Hospitals usually arrange for a nurse to carry your baby to the car. Your husband must not rush you. Your stitches may not let you walk at a normal pace, and if you have had a Caesarean section you can only walk very slowly indeed.

When you get home, a competent husband will have already cleared up a bit, removing dirty dishes from the table and empty milk (or other) bottles from the kitchen. He will have guessed that you will not want to be faced with a scene suggesting that you now have the task of looking after two dependants. He will certainly not have organised a reception party. In winter (or even in summer) he will have turned up the central heating so that, for the first day or two, the house approaches the temperature of the hospital, probably about 72°F (22°C). It can then be turned down a degree every day until your usual house temperature is reached.

You might want to have a cup of coffee in the kitchen and generally settle back into being at home again (this does not mean washing the kitchen floor). Sooner or later, change back into a nightie or pyjamas and pile into bed with the baby by your side. Start as you mean to continue by contracting your pelvic floor while you lie in bed resolving to do 50 a day in groups of five. Work out a way of reminding yourself about these for the next two days – a Post-it sticky note on your alarm clock/changing trolley/crib, for instance.

Quite possibly you will feel unreal and in a dream which can be somewhat unsettling. This is common, is called depersonalisation, and is nothing to get fussed about. There isn't much that you have to do at this stage except be there for your baby. The feeling will wear off after a day or two.

A feeling of exhaustion can wash over you at any stage, especially if you are anaemic. Normally, a healthy woman has blood with a haemoglobin level of 12 to 14 grams per 100 ml. Haemoglobin is the red pigment in blood that transports oxygen around the body. Loss of blood during birth and afterwards will leave you anaemic with a low haemoglobin level (thin blood) and depleted iron supplies. This is particularly likely after a Caesarean. The hospital will have checked your blood for anaemia before you go home and if necessary will give you iron pills to take. These work over a period of weeks before they are fully effective. You will feel seriously steamrollered if your haemoglobin is below 10 grams per 100 ml.

On the other hand, some new mothers have a manic buzz at this stage and feel they can take on the world. Having been told (or read!) that they will be tired, they are on a high that it is clearly not happening to them. It's a great feeling but a bit of a nuisance because they can't sleep and tend to take on too much. It settles after a few days, or sometimes as long as a couple of weeks.

(STEP-)BROTHERS AND SISTERS

If you have other children, they will want to come and see you and the new baby. Try not to introduce him to them while you are feeding – it can wind them up if they think they have been displaced in your affections. If the baby has brought them a present (see page 60), now is the right time for them to have it. Make sure that you have time to talk to them and listen to their questions or accounts of what they have been doing. Tell them you will be resting in bed for several days. Let them hold the baby if they want to but make it absolutely clear that there is a rule that children are *not allowed to pick up the baby* unless an adult is present.

REST

Try to carry on wearing a nightie or pyjamas and be in or around your bed for the first few days after coming home, however wonderful and exuberant you may feel. This will at least remind other people that you have just had a baby. The old lying-in period was a good principle because it made you move into the slow lane. This is where you want to be for your own sake and in order to fall into step with your baby. Trying to demonstrate to the world that you have not been defeated by giving birth is actually foolish. You need a restful time in order for your body to heal and recuperate from the physical stresses of labour and delivery. Your body also has to adjust to its new, non-pregnant state and to the task of producing milk.

At the same time you have to settle into the patterns and techniques of feeding over the next fortnight or so (see pages 108–12 for more details). This is particularly important if you are breast feeding; if you take the time to get it right now, particularly ensuring an adequate supply of milk, things will be considerably less fraught in a month's time when life hots up a bit. Future success depends on taking it gently now when you and your baby are relatively relaxed so that you can allow the flow of milk to establish itself and you and your baby to get into the same rhythm. Over-enthusiasm messes this up. Hyperactive mothers will find it difficult to settle their babies into successful breast feeding.

At the same time, your baby needs time to recuperate from the massive physiological changes which occur at birth. New babies are generally fairly quiet for the first three weeks and most spend much of their time asleep, especially if they are jaundiced. This is their way of warding off too much stimulation which could make them jittery. The last thing they want at this stage is to be passed around a circle of admirers or be overstimulated by parents entering them for the developmental Olympics. They need some space for themselves and so do you. Don't be misled into thinking that this 'good' phase will necessarily last but do make the most of it.

Let your husband do the fetching and carrying, let him answer the door to callers, telemessages and flowers. He can take the phone calls and organise the meals. It is times like this when the microwave and the take-away come into their own – but beware the way very spicy foods, particularly garlic, can find their way into your breast milk and thus into the baby which makes some babies uncomfortable and restless.

Staying in and around the bedroom will not necessarily guarantee you get sufficient sleep. Your husband must ensure you do get as much as possible. It is in his interests that you do so since the more sleep you get now, the quicker you will recover in the long term. He may have to press you to think of yourself – which is not always easy. New mothers tend to be primarily preoccupied with their babies ('primary maternal preoccupation') and will tend to put their babies' comfort and welfare before their own. They are exquisitely sensitive to their own babies and will be roused by the smallest whimper. This can get out of hand and leave a new mother exhausted.

Fortunately, new babies are comparatively quiet for their first three weeks of life though they are commonly fussier at home than in hospital. At some stage during the day, a good husband will take the baby downstairs and out of your earshot so that you can sleep undisturbed. He should take the phone off the hook and think about putting a Post-it sticky note on the front door asking callers not to ring the bell.

VISITORS

You will be visited every day for a week by a community midwife if you had a normal delivery and for ten days if you had a Caesarean section. This will be at least one new face and possibly several if the community midwives work as a team. They will check that your uterus is contracting down to its original size and inspect your stitches to ensure they are healing well. They will also weigh your baby and check his cord site as well as answering any questions you have. The community midwives are wonderfully calming and reassuring.

The midwife cannot guarantee to call at a particular time so it is helpful to have someone else around in the house to answer the door if you are sleeping or feeding. If this is not possible, put a Post-it sticky note on the door yourself to let people know that you can't answer it.

Other visitors such as family and friends are easier to organise – give them times to call. The same principles apply as did in hospital. Not too many at once and not for too long. Don't feel you have to leap around playing the ultra-competent hostess; they can sort themselves out and are probably pleased to be of practical help. You might even ask them to do some shopping for you.

WHERE WILL THE BABY GO?

For much of the day, he will be beside you, either by your bed or in the kitchen while you are eating. He needs to be adequately warm without being roasted and in general terms he will need one more layer of clothing than you. To gauge how warm he is, slip your hand inside his vest to feel his body temperature or feel the back of his neck. Don't rely on feeling his hands and feet, which in tiny babies are quite often colder than the rest of the body. Babies should never get so hot that they sweat.

You will get a great deal of advice on the question of where he sleeps at night. Perhaps we can recap. You can put him in a cot or crib by your bed, in the bathroom, in his own bedroom or in the nursery in the West Wing. It doesn't matter so long as it is where you feel is right for you and right for him. The only place that is wrong is somewhere with which you don't feel comfortable, even if you have been told it is the right place. He will probably spend most of the day in bed with you but be just a little cautious about keeping him in bed with you through the night because of the risk of him overheating.

The first night at home with a new baby often feels a bit hairy. Remember that *babies are parent-proof* and it is virtually impossible for you to do anything wrong. Go to bed and go to sleep early. Unless your husband has unwisely drunk too much, the perfect man will wake with you for feeds. He can usefully bring you up a cup of tea and a snack as required. Make the most of all this; it is not guaranteed to last, especially when he is back at work. Don't even think of dieting, no matter how flabby you are.

Babies don't always make it easy for you and may choose their first night out of all other options to refuse to settle after a feed. This may be because you had celebratory champagne which a number of babies don't seem to like (claret is better because of its iron content). If he cries instead of settling after a feed, assume it is wind. His father should pick him up and walk him round for fifteen minutes or so rubbing his back to wind him. If this doesn't work, he should try wrapping him up reasonably tightly and putting him down, rhythmically joggling his crib or basket, again for at least fifteen minutes. If all else fails, he will have to walk him round the room over his shoulder for as long as it takes.

Most parents start off with the baby sleeping in their room with them for the first few weeks and then move him into his own room. The usual stimulus for the move is when his snuffling and grunting (and then its episodic cessation) becomes so intrusive that you cannot sleep yourselves.

The night temperature of the room where your baby sleeps should be neither too low nor oven-like. About 66°F (20°C) is sensible. This is warmer than most adults like (another reason why babies are eventually moved into their own rooms) and you will need a convector heater or electric radiator, with a thermostat which can regulate itself, to put in the room where your baby sleeps at night. This is preferable to running your central heating all night. Although your baby will need to be warm, there are real dangers if he overheats. Unlike an older child, he cannot rearrange his duvet or stick a bare foot out from under the covers to cool himself.

It is also a good idea to replace the light bulb or light switch of whichever room he sleeps in with a very low wattage bulb (8 to 15 watts) or a dimmer switch. This is not so you can leave the light on low throughout the night (babies need periods of darkness to help them sleep in the same way as we do) but it prevents your baby from suffering the blinding flash when you switch on the light as you walk in. With a dimmer switch you can turn it half on. If you are really trying, combine the two approaches: a dimmer switch for a main light with a 60 to 100 watt bulb (so that you can look for dropped dummies, etc.) and a table light with a dim bulb for night feeds. Large supermarkets stock 8 watt bulbs.

You will have to feed him at night and will need an extra supply of pillows against which to rest if you are feeding him in your own bed. If he sleeps separately from you and you find you prefer to give the night feeds in his room, you will need to organise a feeding chair and pillows there and have spare nappy-changing gear to hand. If you are breast feeding, you are likely to find yourself thirsty (and probably hungry) while feeding, so it may be sensible to lay in appropriate provisions in advance.

IN WHAT POSITION SHOULD THE BABY SLEEP?

On his back or, if he really will not stay like that, on his side. The important thing is to get him into a habit of sleeping on his back if you can. This cuts down the (tiny) risk of cot death in later weeks. If he will only settle on his side, put him down on a different side each time you pick him up. Do not put him down to sleep on his front. Cot deaths have been cut dramatically since mothers were advised not to put young babies to sleep on their fronts. This makes sense in any case because he will spend much of the time at this stage curled up and won't straighten out to sleep face-down that readily. He was in this flexed position before he was born and will feel most comfortable this way.

Place your baby with his feet near the end of the Moses basket or carrycot, so if he manages to wriggle he won't disappear under his top blanket.

Small babies feel more secure if they are swaddled and this also helps stabilise their temperature. Wrap a flannelette or brushed cotton (Winceyette) receiving/swaddling sheet around the baby including his shoulders and arms. This shouldn't be too tight – the purpose is essentially to make him feel more secure. If your baby sucks his fingers, leave the appropriate arm outside so he can do so.

YOUR BABY

During this first week he will come out in white spots over his nose and upper cheeks. These are milia. They are sometimes called milk spots, which is misleading as they have nothing to do with the quality or type of milk the baby is having. They are *normal* and will go of their own accord. Do not pick or squeeze them.

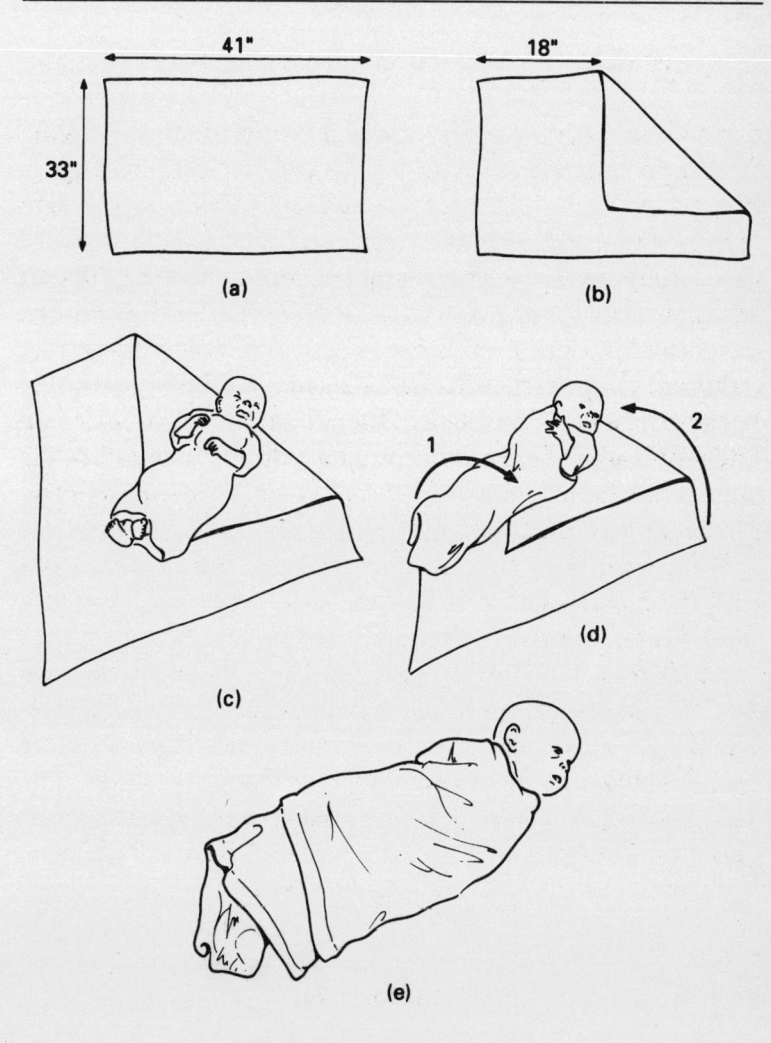

Figure 9 Swaddling a baby

Within the week, the stump of the umbilical cord drops off (to the great relief of most mothers). Occasionally it hangs on until the end of the second week, in which case you must keep on with the routine for cleaning it which you were shown in hospital, however squeamish you may feel. It is a potential site for bacterial infection which can track up to the baby's liver. Once the cord has dropped off, no special cleaning procedure is necessary.

Tiny babies have long fingernails and will scratch their own faces. Don't be afraid to cut the nails using baby scissors – it's easier than the traditional practice of nibbling them. Hiccups and sneezes are common and of no particular significance. Some sneezes are triggered by bright light.

You may notice that your baby sometimes has a squint which, if it comes and goes, doesn't usually matter at this stage. It is most likely to be a result of him not yet having learned to coordinate his eye movements. A permanent squint needs investigating. An eye infection with sticky eyelids and a discharge is something to mention to your midwife. Meanwhile, bathe the eye with sterile water (boiled water that has been cooled), wiping from the tear duct to the outside of the eye. Change the cotton wool pad for the other eye. A non-conventional treatment which often works, having done the above, is to drop a little of your breast milk into his eye.

At approximately seven days (unless it has been done in hospital), a community midwife will prick the baby's heel to take a tiny amount of blood for a Guthrie test and thyroid hormone level. This is a routine measure to check that your baby does not have phenylketonuria or hypothyroidism. Both are rare conditions causing retarded development.

FEEDING GENERALLY

With luck, you and your baby will be getting into the swing of things. He may get back to birth weight by the end of the first week though the average baby will not do this until ten days (and therefore some will take longer).

By now, bottle-fed babies will be feeding approximately four-hourly and taking the amounts recommended on the packet. Breast-fed babies don't settle into a routine nearly so easily; it takes some time for your breasts and your baby between them to establish enough milk at each feed.

All babies are different and, after a week or so, most mothers are pretty good at sussing out their own baby's feeding requirements. This means they will be getting to know how often and for how long they need to feed in order for their baby to thrive.

You can expect your baby to have a wet nappy at least once a day but the frequency of bowel movements varies enormously in breast-fed babies. Bottle-fed babies open their bowels daily. A baby who does not feed can get dehydrated and not pass urine daily. If you think this is the case, point it out to your midwife who can check his state of hydration by seeing if his fontanelle is slack and alerting your doctor accordingly. Another time to alert your midwife is if the usual yellowish stool turns green.

BREAST FEEDING

If you are breast feeding, it helps to keep certain principles in mind.

Supply and demand

The breast will produce as much milk as is removed from it. Effectively it has a memory for how much milk is needed. Demand produces supply. If the breast is not producing enough (your baby doesn't settle after a feed and is not putting on enough weight), feed your baby more often so that more milk is removed. More will then be produced. If a hungry baby is given a supplementary bottle (or if he is given a bottle at night), he will be less hungry and empty the breast less well at his next feed. The breast will then produce less milk. With less milk available, the baby will be hungry and need a supplementary bottle. At the next feed, he will not be so hungry and take less from the breast ... and so on. Be very careful about supplementary bottle feeds if you are breast feeding – the breast has no way of knowing that it has not produced enough milk and doesn't realise that it should produce more.

Technique

If necessary, ask for advice and supervision from someone who knows her business – a midwife, health visitor or feeding counsellor. Be wary of reading too many books at a time – they tend to contradict themselves.

Take the trouble to find a comfortable position for feeding. If you and your baby are comfortable, a feed is much more likely to go well. You are also going to be feeding your baby for several months so if you get into good postural habits during these early days you will help prevent future shoulder and back problems. If you are sitting in a chair to feed, there are some important points:

- Sit with your bottom well back so the small of your back is supported by the chair – if you like, tuck a small cushion behind your waist.
- Take your baby to the breast rather than the breast to your baby. This means you are likely to need your foot on a stool or a couple of books and the baby on a pillow on your lap.
- Drop your shoulders and relax when he has started to suckle.

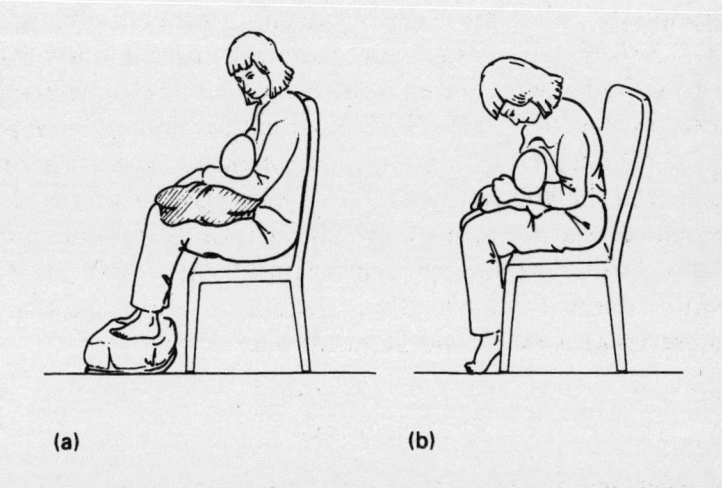

Figure 10 Sitting position for breast feeding: (a) correct (b) wrong

Timing

Don't get obsessed about times. At this stage your priorities are to get your milk supply established which means producing the right amount for your baby. During their first week, most babies over 7 pounds (3.2 kg) in weight will need to be fed about every three to four hours during the day and every four to five hours at night (a total of between six and eight feeds a day). In the interests of ensuring a good milk supply, he will need a minimum of six feeds during a 24-hour period, so do not leave him longer than six hours at night without feeding him during this first week. Smaller and very wakeful babies might need more frequent feeds.

Provided your baby suckles continuously, try not to feed for longer than 20 minutes each side. A baby is able to take most of the milk he needs in the first five minutes when his suck is strongest. This means that a baby who feeds for much longer than fifteen minutes each side is spending much of the time sucking for pleasure, not milk – he is using the nipple as a dummy. In actual fact, most people manage with ten minutes each side starting with a different breast on each occasion.

Forget about routines but don't fall into the trap of putting a fussy baby to the breast every twenty minutes because it pacifies him. He won't be feeding so much as sucking for comfort or for the hell of it and you will be making a rod for your own back. Try other ways of comforting him like rocking, pacing, singing or giving him a dummy (see page 116–17). So-called demand feeding does not mean whipping out a breast at every whinge from the baby. It means feeding the baby when he is hungry rather than making him wait the next 34 minutes because that is in his routine schedule. In any case, you can't impose a routine until you are producing enough milk for your baby.

COMMON BREAST-FEEDING PROBLEMS

Sore nipples

This is, in our experience, the commonest reason for giving up breast feeding. There are rather too many theories about the causes of sore nipples though poor latching on is well recognised. We have also been struck by the escalating number of mothers with sore nipples occurring since it has been declared fashionable to encourage the baby to suckle for protracted periods in the first few days.

First aid in case of sore nipples is as follows:

- Put your baby to the breast at a different angle e.g. 'football' hold, with his body and legs under your arm rather than across your lap (see page 156–7).
- Take two paracetamol in water at least half an hour before feeding. (This, of course, is very much easier in theory than in practice!)
- Feed on the less painful nipple first (forget starting on alternating sides for the time being).
- Try feeding your baby through a nipple shield.
- Don't let your baby suck longer than ten minutes at each breast.
- Make sure that he is latching on and you are disconnecting him from the breast properly.

Most sore nipples are just suffering from unaccustomed wear but this may progress to a cracked nipple ('wear and tear') which is extraordinarily painful and can bleed so you see blood in the baby's mouth. Some creams can be helpful but don't go mad. What really helps healing is allowing the nipple to dry gently, which in practice means exposing your breasts to the air. On the occasions that it is not appropriate for you to go topless, a useful trick is to put a tea strainer (handle removed) into your bra to hold the material away from the nipple and allow air to circulate. What you don't want is your nipple wallowing in soggy breast pads, especially not those with a plastic backing.

If things get too bad, contact your local feeding counsellor or NCT branch and allow an electric breast pump (which is actually not painful) to empty the affected breast while you carry on feeding with the other breast – at least until the other nipple packs up through over-use. You can avoid this by putting the expressed (pumped) breast milk in a bottle for your baby and trying to get him to feed from the bottle. Playtex bottles have teats which are most like human nipples. Even then, he might not take from it, just to add to your problems, in which case rejoice in the fact that you at least have a sense of humour.

Not enough milk?

This has nothing to do with breast size. As a first step, *do not* resort to supplementary bottles. Try offering more frequent feeds on the basis that the more your breasts are emptied, the more milk they will produce. (There is a time lag of two or three days before the breasts get the message and respond by producing more milk though, so be patient.) You will need to offer at least two extra feeds in a 24-hour period, so you will probably have to wake your baby to feed him.

Your baby doesn't suck

This may be because you have an unusual nipple shape or your nipple is inverted. In such circumstances you need expert, individual attention from an experienced midwife or feeding counsellor to help your baby latch on. Occasionally, babies seem to have very short tongues which make matters difficult for them.

A baby with oral thrush (infection with candida) will have a sore mouth and may be in two minds about sucking. This is not a serious condition and can be easily treated by your general practitioner.

In the first week or so, jaundiced babies are often drowsy and have to be coaxed by withdrawing the nipple when they stop sucking. Massaging their feet or stroking under their chin when they stop sucking also helps them start up again.

BOTTLE FEEDING

The good thing about bottle feeding is its sheer flexibility and the freedom it gives you to sleep through the night and go out during the day or evening. It is also easier to master. Apart from the general principles of keeping things sterile, the only other likely complication is technical troubles with the teat. It should deliver one drop a second when the bottle is held upside down – make a bigger hole with a red-hot needle if it doesn't.

You need not feed so frequently with a bottle as formula milk takes longer than breast milk to digest. Keep things sterile and don't use bottle warmers as they breed bacteria. Most people use a microwave but be very careful to *shake the bottle well after heating* as it will have been warmed unevenly. Microwave ovens can produce 'hot-spots' in milk that can burn unless they have been dispersed by shaking. *Always check the temperature* by allowing a few drops to fall on the inside of your wrist before offering the bottle to the baby. You are checking that it is not too hot – some babies are quite happy with cold milk and it makes no nutritional difference.

It is relatively easy to overfeed a bottle-fed baby. Measure quantities carefully (no more powder than recommended) and don't insist he finishes the bottle. As with breast feeding, be guided by his weight gain (4 to 7 oz or 120 to 210 grams a week after birth weight is restored). There isn't as much difference between different milks as you might think. A midwife or health visitor can advise you, but don't get into soya without the supervision of your general practitioner or paediatrician because its nutritional balance is different.

Remember that bottle-fed babies can get thirsty. If he seems hungry between feeds yet is gaining weight well,

116 YOUR NEW BABY

offer him boiled (not boiling) water or specially prepared baby juices (some people use dilute camomile tea specially prepared and packaged for babies).

DUMMIES

Unfortunately these are unfashionable at present and often evoke cries of horror. However, dummies can be indispensable in the early weeks, especially if you have a 'sucky'

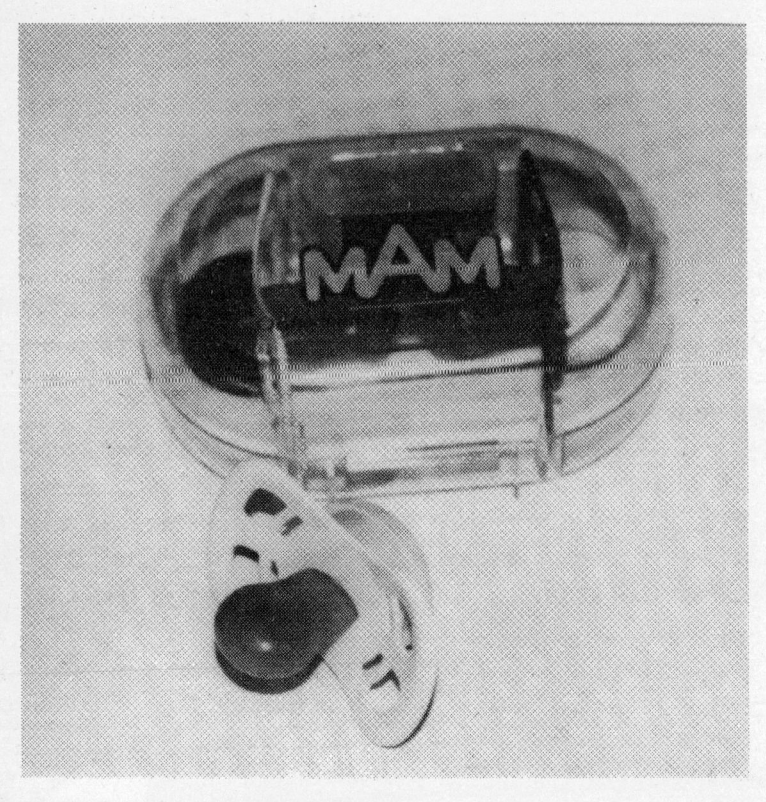

Figure 11 Mini-Mam dummy

or unsettled baby. Now is the time to try one when he is trying to get to sleep. There is absolutely nothing wrong in letting a small baby do what he enjoys – sucking – so long as he doesn't do it all the time. In any case, virtually all parents would agree there is nothing worse than a crying baby. A dummy helps a baby to learn a self-soothing behaviour. Used judiciously he won't get dependent on it and demand it all the time.

Giving a baby a dummy to help him settle himself does not mean you will have a two-year-old plugged in, neither does it mean you will ruin your child's future tooth formation (ask any orthodontist). Buy an orthodontic shaped teat designed for babies under six months. A firm called Mini-Mam produce just this type which has the further advantage of not having a huge ring on it for the baby to catch his fingers in and pull out accidentally. Don't tie the dummy on with a string around his neck. You can throw the dummy away when your baby is about four or five months old. By this time, he will have developed interests beyond just sucking, and you will be feeling more in control of things.

STAGE 4

Life in the slow and middle lanes

14

One to three weeks: life in the slow lane

With any luck your baby will still be relatively quiet for the next couple of weeks. This period, up to when your baby is three weeks old, is a time for you to continue to recover physically from labour and birth and for you and your baby to settle into getting to know each other. Live your life in the slow lane. If you are breast feeding, it is also the time to continue to get the feeding established. All this will be accomplished most successfully if you remain quietly at home. Nipping into the office followed by a quick dash round the supermarket will neither help your episiotomy to heal nor your milk supply to flourish.

If your husband has managed to take three or four days off work to see you and your baby back home and get you established, he will now have gone back to work. He can hand over to your mother who might move in if that is what suits you both. It is important that you eat properly – this means breakfast, a decent lunch (not a diet yoghurt and a Mars bar) and supper – and having someone at home is often helpful in ensuring you eat meals. However, your husband should certainly not expect you to be bouncing around conjuring up tasty evening meals and there is still no way you are going to host a drinks party. He needs to come home promptly from work and avoid the temptation to linger with his mates. You (and his baby) come first.

If your husband has been able to negotiate formal paternity leave, his job is to help you to stay in the slow lane. He should take on some housework, the shopping and the general organisation of household chores. This means planning meals and their preparation in advance, rather than hovering around looking for an opportunity to be useful. It is possible that he may need some guidance – for example, your evening meal needs to be earlier than he might think. Not many women at this stage are going to want to be hanging around for the four-course gourmet meal at 9.30 p.m.

You will by now be feeling slightly less dazed and a little more capable. You will still need to get as much sleep as you can. Much of your waking day is going to be spent in feeding, changing and washing the baby. Take things more slowly than you would usually; don't rush anything, as you still won't feel very organised. Plan no more than one social activity a day. A friend for coffee and your mother-in-law for tea may well be too much. People who haven't had babies can be a bit of a problem; see only a few of them. As they have not experienced primary maternal preoccupation themselves, they do not realise that you are in your own time capsule. They may not understand why you hadn't noticed that World War III had broken out yesterday, or why you don't care if it has. They will go home saying to their friends, 'We've lost her. Can't think of anything but the baby. Talk about vague. She's completely knocked off.'

Keep cuddling your baby (of course!). You will have to

wake him up if necessary every four hours for a feed but don't keep prodding and fiddling with him when he is resting. Talk to him and laugh with him when he is alert but don't be too impatient to have major fun with him; he needs a quiet couple of weeks to adapt to the outside world. Keep him swaddled and lying on his back or side. He will still have a floppy head which needs support when you pick him up. If you give him to other people to hold (and you probably won't want to do too much of that), remind them to put their fingers behind his head if you think they are unused to babies. Don't remind your mother unless you want to elicit a short lecture from her about her own extensive child-rearing competence.

Try to nudge both yourself and your baby towards a regular afternoon nap. If you have a baby who never seems to sleep when you are able to, try putting him into bed with you. If you are in bed together, you know he is safe and you may manage to get a nap even if he doesn't. If you have someone at home with you, it's clearly their role to take your baby for an hour or two in the afternoon so you can go to bed. Have an afternoon rest even if you don't feel like going to sleep.

After the first week home, the community midwife hands over to the health visitor who will probably ring or visit and get to know both you and your baby. The health visitor will have been a midwife herself as part of her training. Find out from her where your local child health clinic is (it might be at your GP's surgery). You will need to take your baby to be weighed there every two weeks, at least for the first few months.

If you haven't been given a Child Health Record in hospital, the health visitor will give you one. This is kept by you and contains entries from any healthcare professionals who have dealings with your baby. It is your baby's medical record and the argument is that it is less likely to be lost if you keep it than if it is consigned to the mercy of a medical records department.

Once your baby has settled in at home, you can reduce the central heating temperature down to its usual level. This may mean that you will want to discard your nightie and get into a track suit when it suits you. You are likely to find it takes you half the day to get dressed in any case. Unhappily, unless you are very lucky, most of your ordinary clothes will still not yet fit. Don't worry – you can deal with that problem later. Depending on the season and the outside temperature, aim for a trip outdoors with the baby when you can face it (this can seem a major hurdle). Discover how to get to the child health clinic or go and register the baby at the local Register Office.

At some stage, before your baby starts to get restless in the evenings (which begins at about three weeks), see if you can get someone to mind the baby while you and your husband scamper out for a quick meal and some time together for each other. You are not only a mother, you are still a wife. But don't let him even contemplate sex yet – you certainly won't. If the topic surfaces, talk about stitches, lochia, clots and, if this fails, techniques of circumcision. Your lochia, incidentally, will now be lessening but the same principle applies as before – if you pass any clots, try to keep them and show the midwife or health visitor.

EXERCISES

Take time to do the postnatal exercises that you were shown in hospital. The most important thing is to carry on with 50 pelvic floor lifts a day. A good way to remember is to do them while you are feeding – five lifts for each breast, or five lifts for the first ounce and five lifts for the last ounce if you are bottle feeding. At this stage you will find that your buttock and/or your abdominal muscles will want to contract at the same time to try and help your weak pelvic floor muscles, so you will need to concentrate on isolating the pelvic floor muscles. This means that when you do a pelvic floor lift no other muscle should move! You can also practise stopping peeing in midstream – eventually you will be able to stop the flow of urine, but for the time being, be content if you can just slow it. There is no need to practise this more than once every few days.

Your abdominal muscles are still likely to be stretched and weak. You may notice, to your dismay, that you *still* look about four to six months' pregnant, especially if you have had a Caesarean section. At this stage, still concentrate on holding your tummy muscles in while you are standing and walking. This will restore the elastic in the muscles, which is necessary before you begin active rehabilitation work. While you are around the house, *don't* cover up the pot belly with a baggy sweater so that you forget about it – wear something that continually reminds you to hold your tummy in. If you have been given an exercise sheet by the hospital, try to do these exercises once a day (but not at the expense of your afternoon rest). See the sheet in Appendix 6 at the end of this book if you haven't already got one (pages 227–8).

If there is a local postnatal exercise class (and sometimes you may be lucky enough to find that your local hospital provides this) get in touch but check out what is involved. Prancing around in a leotard is simply not on at this stage. You might find that there is a postnatal support group in the area which is a different sort of thing and allows a group of new mothers to make friends and gas to one another. If you went to an antenatal class you might like to make a few phone calls to other class members to see if they have had their babies yet. You won't feel quite so much on your own if you can rabbit on to each other about how things have been and how things are, but don't get competitive about your babies' feeding and sleeping patterns.

FEEDING (AND VOMITING)

You and your baby should still be settling into a feeding rhythm that suits you both if you are breast feeding, whereas if you are bottle feeding, you will probably have got it licked. With any luck you will be feeling much more relaxed about feeding times and be more comfortable about shifting your position as you feed. You will also have had time to organise appropriate chairs with pillows and foot stools, so that everywhere you feed your baby you can sit with the top half of your body relaxed and your shoulders at the same height as each other.

One particular problem which may crop up is the baby vomiting. Roughly speaking there are three patterns to this.

Some babies, mainly those that are breast-fed, seem greedy and positively gulp down their feed which then bounces back. This is probably because milk can flow more freely from the nipple than it can from the teat of a bottle.

Although a baby has to suck to obtain milk from a bottle, some breasts produce a flow of milk which positively spurts and overwhelms a small baby's capacity to deal with it.

Other babies are just sicky babies and 'posset' small quantities of milk every time they are picked up. It drives their mothers to distraction yet there is absolutely nothing to worry about apart from the smell that lingers on your clothes. After a while you get used to carrying around a muslin square (puke rag) with you and putting it on anyone's shoulder if they are going to hold the baby. The amount they bring up always looks more than it actually is and it is extremely unlikely that the baby will starve. Mothers frequently worry about this type of baby vomiting but, if the baby is putting on weight, it is *very unlikely* there is anything seriously wrong. Comfort yourself by the thought that it will stop at about the time they start to crawl (and if you want to discomfort yourself, consider that crawling starts at about seven months).

Don't put sicky babies or greedy babies on their backs immediately after a feed unless you are in the room with them because of the remote danger that they might choke on their own vomit. Wait 20 minutes before leaving them on their own or put them on their side to begin with.

A few, mainly boy babies, develop projectile vomiting which means that they can eject a stream of vomit for nearly a metre. The house acquires a new aroma after a week or two. Such vomiting usually interferes with the baby's weight gain, but in any case you should consult your GP sooner rather than later as the cause may be pyloric stenosis. This is an uncommon physical condition which prevents the stomach from emptying properly. It will need treatment.

If your baby catches a cold he may vomit because he is swallowing mucus. Incidentally, a baby catches a cold because of a virus, not because he has an incompetent mother who left him in a draught or who took him for a walk and got caught in the rain. Colds are a problem before the age of six weeks because a tiny baby finds it difficult to breathe through his mouth. This is frightening for the parents. He also finds feeding with a blocked-up nose difficult and quickly tires. Yet babies must keep their fluid intake up, particularly if they have a temperature. This means more frequent, short feeds for a breast-fed baby, and water offered between feeds for a bottle-fed baby. You can temporarily kiss goodbye to any pattern of feeding which may have been emerging. Keep your baby in the same room as you and don't let him overheat. A room humidifier (Pifco make a good one) will help keep his nose unblocked and enable him to breathe more easily. If his snot turns green, if he goes off his food, or if you are worried, call your GP.

CHANGING NAPPIES

You must remember to look after yourself, particularly your back. As you now know, it is very common for new mothers to develop low back pain at some stage but you can reduce the chance of it happening to you. Make sure you have a surface which is at your *waist height* on which to change your baby's nappy. You will be changing your baby as often as ten times a day at this stage and you will get low backache if the changing mat is too low. Block the changing trolley up on books or telephone directories if necessary to bring it to the correct height for you. (If the trolley has castors, you will obviously need to unscrew them first.) It is also useful to keep a low stool 8–9 inches high or a thick book under the changing table so you can rest a foot on it while changing your baby. This stops you arching your lower back.

Don't change him on the bed without kneeling on the floor. A changing mat helps avoid any mess or spills but you ideally need two: one for upstairs and one downstairs. If you only have one, remember that there is no point in

(a)   (b)

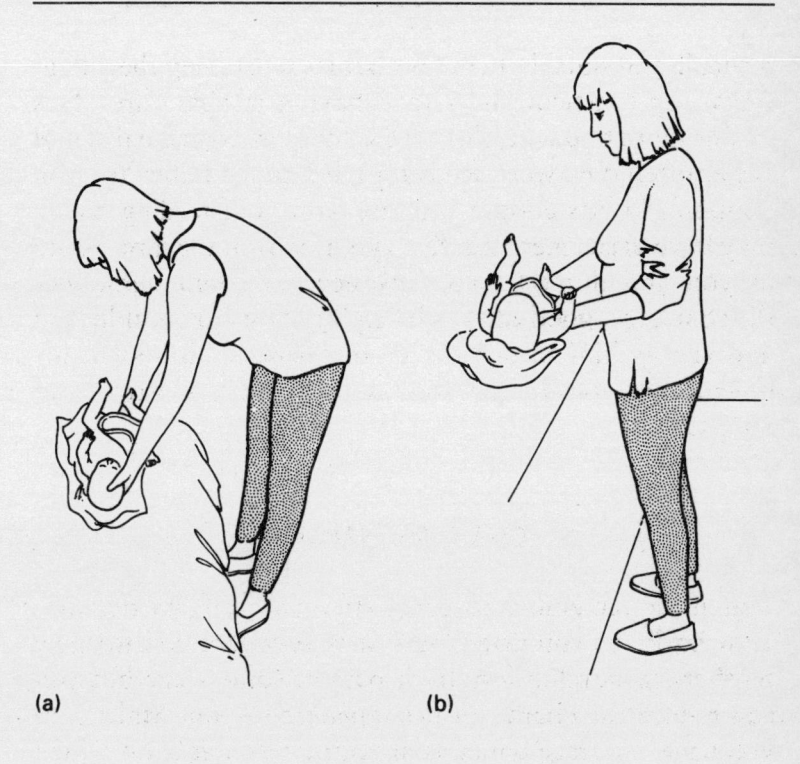

Figure 12 Changing baby: (a) wrong (b) correct

you carrying your baby up a flight of stairs (especially if you have had a Caesarean section) just to whip off a damp nappy. The kitchen table will do. Cover your plastic changing mat with a muslin nappy to shield the baby from the touch of chilly vinyl. The muslin will also soak up the inevitable jet of urine which will otherwise trickle on to the floor.

It is easier to change your baby near running water. Breast-fed babies have fairly odourless stools but those who are bottle fed can put out some stinkers. If your baby has passed a stool, clean his bottom with warm water, using your hand or cotton wool. Some authorities caution against the use of soap, but Simple soap (the trade name for soap that has absolutely no additives) in our experience causes no problems. Alternatively you can use baby wipes or lotion to clean the buttocks, and run the small risk of a temporary local allergic reaction developing. After drying his bottom, put some barrier cream (basic zinc and castor oil or Sudocrem) on his buttocks. This is the most potent protection against nappy rash, the main cause of which tends to be leaving a baby to lounge around in a soggy nappy. Introduce your husband to the joys of nappy changing sooner rather than later and praise his prowess, irrespective of your private judgement.

WASHING AND BATHING

You will have to clean your baby's bottom every time he has a dirty nappy. He won't need a bath every day but you will need to do the following each day – wipe both eyes using a separate piece of wet cotton wool for each. Soap under his chin, under his armpits and behind his ears. Pat dry these areas carefully – they can sometimes get sore. He might need some E45 cream behind his ears which can get quite crusted and unhealthy looking.

If you are going to give him a bath on his own, be very careful to go down on one knee rather than bending over while standing. The best baby baths are those which hook over the side of your bath, fill from your bath taps and have their own plug. This means that the baby is at a reasonable level and you don't have to lug gallons of water around. Watch out for the water temperature – always check it yourself by putting a dry hand or elbow in.

The easiest and most fun way to bath a baby is to put him into the adult bath with his father. The water can be

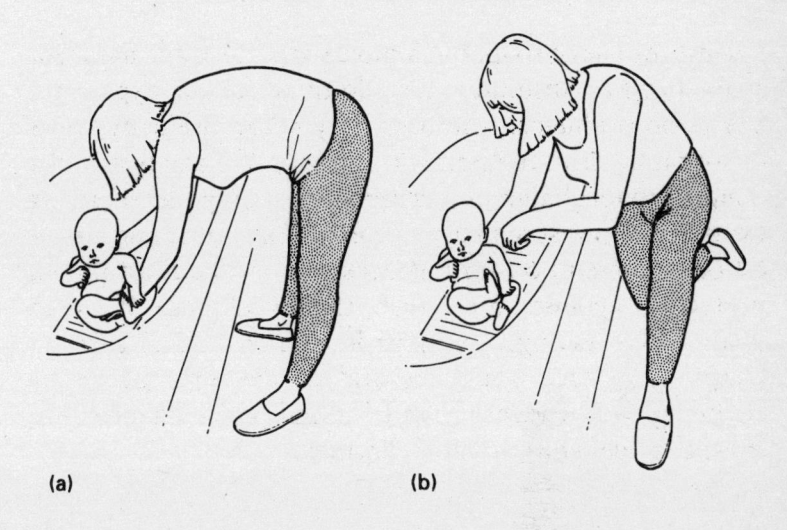

Figure 13 Bathing baby: (a) wrong (b) correct

the usual comfortable temperature for most adults (assuming they don't like it as hot as it is possible to tolerate) and the procedure is enjoyable rather than a chore. When you lift him (the baby) out, wrap him quickly in his own towel, warmed if possible.

Dry his umbilicus but don't tip powder into it. You can still bath a baby if his cord is determined to stay attached. If you have been shown a cleaning routine for the stump, use this when you have dried him. If you have not, simply pat it dry without showering powder on it.

Brush his hair daily and keep an eye open for cradle cap (crusty scales) which will need to be anointed with any of several lotions you can buy and subsequently can be worked off with a very soft toothbrush or nailbrush.

15

Three to six weeks: life in the middle lane

At two to three weeks many babies start to come out of the rather dozy ('good') state they have been in up to now. In particular they come to life in the evenings, often quite noisily. Their previously quiet demeanour has helped shield them from too much stimulation too early but now they're getting ready for it (even if you aren't). As they warm up, their individual personality or temperament becomes more clearly defined. It is now that your baby begins to take an active interest in the world around him. His eyes seek out complex patterns. Your face is still the most fascinating thing as far as he is concerned but mobiles and musical toys are beginning to stake their claim and can be cautiously deployed. Be a little wary of overstimulation and producing a jittery baby by throwing too many toys and excitements at him too soon.

Day by day he is becoming physically more robust and noticeably bigger. His face may have broken out in unattractive spots which should be ignored. They will go after a week or two. Just occasionally this is exacerbated by using too much washing powder for his sheets. You may be concerned that he does not defaecate every day but breast-fed babies often don't. A baby is not constipated unless his stools are hard.

At the same time, three weeks of interrupted nights are catching up with you and you will feel less robust. Any manic buzz will have worn off and it is likely that you are now feeling somewhat drained. Nevertheless, you have to rise to the occasion and cope with an increasingly demanding baby. At some stage in the next three weeks your mother and any maternity nurse will both have gone, possibly leaving you with a crisis of confidence. Don't set yourself too high a standard. Your task at this stage is to survive. Sit it out; it gets better in time.

For most of the day now you will be up in day clothes and pottering around. The pace of life moves into the middle lane. The days change little but you can expect the evenings to become a strain. From three weeks on (allow proportionally longer for a premature baby) comforting your baby in the evening burns up a great deal of time. You will find yourself developing new expertise in pacing up and down, jiggling the baby and singing softly into his ear. Your husband gets used to coming home to the sound of grizzling baby and you both get used to having the baby with you at supper.

You will not yet be physically perfect! Your lochia will have started to tail off and turn progressively browner. It will stop at about five weeks. Meanwhile your stitches will be dissolving, and you may find what look like little worms on your pad as they break up and come away. Continue your pelvic floor exercises – *this is a priority*. You should still be aiming for 50 contractions a day in groups of five and hopefully will have programmed yourself to do them while feeding. You should find by now that you can slow (or even stop) the flow of urine midstream more efficiently.

Now that you have mastered quick pelvic floor contractions ('flicks'), introduce one extra exercise. Concentrating on the vagina, contract the pelvic floor as usual, but *hold* the contraction for as long as you can. Try initially to sustain the contraction for a slow count of six. If this presents no problem, and the muscle fibres haven't started to relax before you want them to, try sustaining the contraction for a count of ten. Your ultimate aim will be to sustain a contraction for a slow count of around 30 by the time your baby is about six months (three months if you had a Caesarean) (see Appendix 7 on pages 229–30). This exercise does more than restore tone; it will actually strengthen your pelvic floor muscles and needs to be added to the quick flicks. Don't despair if, in spite of masses of pelvic floor exercises, your muscles still don't seem to respond very well. It is still early days and if you had a long or difficult second stage of labour probably involving forceps (especially Kielland's) it is going to take longer for your pelvic floor muscles to recover. They will!

Continue doing the abdominal exercises described on your hospital sheet if you were given one: otherwise the best book to buy is *The Postnatal Exercise Book* by Margie Polden and Barbara Whiteford (London, Frances Lincoln Ltd).

Most women will not be thinking of sex yet, except with apprehension. If you have already had sex, that's great. You won't have done any damage (but unless you were careful you may now be pregnant again!).

YOUR BABY'S PERSONALITY

Everyone who has had more than one baby knows that each baby is different. Not just in appearance but in the whole way in which they go about their lives, their general style. Some have a sunny disposition, others are more irritable. Some are placid, others excitable. The sort of style your baby has is pivotal for your morale as a new parent.

The crucial thing to grasp is that *babies are different* right from the word go. Anyone who has worked with a number of newborn babies will tell you this is obvious. They are born with a particular personality or temperamental style in place and start off life with it. It doesn't mean they stay like that for ever. Early temperament is not by any means fixed and will change gradually over months and years according to their experiences and how they are handled. In other words, the personality of any developing child is a combination of what he was born with and what he has experienced subsequently.

It gets a little more complicated. How your baby is in terms of personality will affect what you do to him. A sunny, placid baby is easy to care for, stresses his parents less, and is therefore more likely to experience a sunny, placid mother. Easy-going babies are easy to look after. They feed easily and with pleasure. They sleep soundly at predictable times. They enjoy novelty and stimulation without getting uncontrollably excited. They can be jollied out of a crying spell. They like people and life in general. They produce a feeling of confidence and affection in those who care for them, so these babies themselves create a surrounding environment which is loving and luxurious. They elicit good experiences for themselves and this helps them acquire feelings of security and confidence. Thus their personality develops positively. They carry on being easy to live with.

In contrast, an irritable baby who is hard to soothe is more likely to make any mother impatient. Babies who are tetchy, irritable, easily upset, continually crying, intolerant of changes in their routine, apparently uncooperative and unpredictable, are hard to live with. Such a style was called 'difficult' in a flash of inspiration by one group of developmental psychologists. They are certainly extremely difficult to look after. What works for such babies on one day winds them up on another. They make their care-givers irritable and uncertain. Thus they unwittingly surround themselves with irritability and unpredictability as their mothers try a number of things in order to find something which will placate them. This is just the sort of situation they cannot tolerate themselves and yet they are very likely to stir it up by the effect they have on others. A vicious spiral develops. Their unfortunate personality style elicits from others just the sort of short-tempered, exasperated handling which *they cannot tolerate*. Their experience of this handling creates in them an apprehension of the world and a feeling of not being secure in it. They grumble, protest and despair openly. This exasperates their parents and so the vicious spiral continues.

Partly, the reason why babies like this are so difficult to care for is obvious. Irritable, quirky people who dislike changes in their lives are more demanding than those who are benign and unflappable. But there is another dimension. Parents tend to look to their children for an indication as to whether they are being good parents. If you have an easy baby who smiles at everything and is adaptable you feel you are doing your job well. But if you have a gritty infant who protests about everything you do to him, you rapidly get the feeling that you are doing something wrong. It feels as though he's letting you know that you are an incompetent parent. You begin to wonder whether you are coping at all. After all, you say to yourself, I should be able to have a smiling, satisfied child all the time, given that I have given him such a perfect start.

Well, actually you can't. No one can. The mother who sets out to anticipate accurately her baby's every need and meet it without compromising principle, personal health or her relationship with her husband will produce an over-indulged, spoilt brat at the end of it. For babies, as for the rest of us, some frustration is necessary in order to stimulate us into developing new ways of coping and new insights (i.e. growing up). Some grit is necessary to produce a pearl (not that the oyster particularly enjoys the process).

In any case, judging your own parenting capacity by looking for short-term results in your child is doomed to failure. The personalities and styles of babies and children are *not* just the result of parental handling. Firstly, as babies are born with different temperamental styles, they already have something on board at the start of things, before any parent has got to them. Secondly, they have other experiences in life apart from those which parents provide. Thirdly, the amount of influence that parents have over their children's personalities is much less than most people (including quite a lot of professionals) think. Most parents provide entirely adequate parenting in the middle range of, for instance, the use of punishment or indulgence. It is the extremes of parenting which affect children's personalities, usually in a damaging way. Even then, most children are proof against their parents. Just think how different siblings are, one from another, in spite of having the same parents. You simply cannot judge your capability as a parent just by looking at your child.

This is particularly important if you have a baby who is excitable, grizzly, hates new things and is irregular in his biological rhythms (so that he doesn't sleep or get hungry at predictable times). This is the classic 'difficult' pattern recognised by child development scientists and which applies to about one baby in ten. Such a baby may take hours to feed, doing so grumpily and protestingly, and then sick it all up again. It will be impossible for you to feel that you are doing a good job. He will cry an enormous amount yet it won't be possible to work out what he is protesting about. Whatever you do doesn't soothe him but if you try something new he hates it. You can never bank on getting a break from things because you don't know when he's going to sleep or soil his nappy. It is a bit of a nightmare because you think you are supposed to be in control but don't feel you are and accuse yourself of failing.

Older and more experienced mothers will say about you 'She's got a difficult one there', just as they might say that about certain difficult husbands – 'I don't know how she puts up with him.' This is true wisdom, acknowledging as it does the role of the baby's inborn temperament. Unfortunately, the common assumption among many young(ish) adults is that your baby is a direct result of your parenting ability alone, that a baby's personality is completely the result of his upbringing. This is naive and wrong. Nevertheless it is a common view. Friends and relatives may jump to the assumption that they could do better and may be tempted to offer advice. It is infuriating and demoralising but remind yourself that *everyone* believes themselves to be an expert when it comes to babies and child development!

Looking after a difficult baby is one of the most trying things anyone has to do. There are few inbuilt rewards and you have to run on good faith that what you are doing is the right thing. To do this you need support, not cheap criticism. If only your friends were to say to you, like a more experienced parent might, 'I don't know how you manage – you're so good with him', then you would feel more supported (so long as you didn't feel they were criticising your baby). They probably won't say anything like that, so you have to say it to yourself and make sure that your husband says it too (and means it). Easy babies make it easy to be a 'good' parent, difficult babies make parents do all the work. And easy babies are more common than difficult ones. Not everyone has had the experience and knows what it is like.

One way of thinking about all this is to recognise that a difficult baby actually lacks certain attributes which have not yet developed in him. He doesn't yet have the capacity to soothe himself which is evident in the easy baby who relaxes easily into sleep after a feed. He lacks the capacity to accept change and be stimulated by novelty. He doesn't possess the self-regulation reflected in a steady rhythmicity of biological functions. He can't seem to know when he is satisfied (so he over-feeds) or know what is required to make him satisfied (so he grumbles continually). This means you have to do all this for him. He will develop these attributes and skills in time but for the moment you have to fill in the gaps. He is exporting his shortcomings into you and you have to rise to the occasion in order to supply him with what he lacks by soothing him, reassuring him and adopting a steady, patient, settled routine.

Because a difficult temperament is largely a reflection of things that have not yet developed (like self-soothing skills), it tends to sort itself out in the longer run as these capacities mature. Even the most difficult baby, if treated with a reasonable (not perfect) degree of sympathetic and affectionate care from a parent who is quite clear that she is in charge, will mellow. The personality of most children changes over their first few years. The risk is that parents lose their nerve and respond to a difficult, demanding baby by trying to gratify and indulge him at every turn. They then lose their self-confidence and feel powerless at the hands of an unappeasable tyrant. This is accompanied by anger and bitterness which is shared by the baby who becomes anxious, confused and therefore even more demanding.

The message is clear. If you have a relatively easy, sunny, tolerant baby, thank your lucky stars. He is making it easy for you to be a confident parent. If you have a difficult, unresponsive, demanding baby, you are being put on your mettle. You need to muster support and carry on with what seems intuitively to you to be good enough parenting. Trust your own judgement and don't listen to his apparent criticism. Look after your own self-respect and don't sell your judgement down the river by too much pandering or thrashing around. Provide some degree of consistency and give him the affection he isn't very good at eliciting from you. You have to supply him with what he lacks himself until he develops the skills for self-adaptation, self-regulation and self-soothing – which he will, so long as you can hang on in there. Ultimately *things will improve*.

COPING WITH A CRYING BABY

Until about six weeks when he starts to smile, a baby only has one method of direct communication which is to cry. Before you have a baby of your own it seems straightforward enough to deal with a crying baby – you find out what the cause is and deal with it. But when you have your own baby, it becomes more difficult: it is often far from clear why he is crying. Furthermore, the crying of your own baby is terribly stressful compared with the crying of someone else's, bad though that may be.

Babies have various different types of cry for different

types of discomfort. Mothers who know their babies well can often tell one sort of cry from another, sensing the difference between, for example, a hunger cry and a pain cry. However, they cannot usually do this for all crying and every mother will have experienced the baby who cries persistently and no one can work out why. He is not hungry, nor is he in obvious pain but he is distressed and inevitably making his parents upset too. There certainly are different patterns of crying but knowing this does not help in such circumstances.

If your baby is crying, you feel impelled to find out why and stop it. Ordinarily, you can review possible causes of hunger, pain, anger and misery quite straightforwardly. But when the crying is excessive or persistent things get complicated because you will have already reviewed the straightforward causes but to no avail. Not knowing why your baby is crying adds significantly to the stress of the situation.

One of the commonest assumptions is that crying at this age is typically caused by wind. Certainly some babies swallow air during feeding and become uncomfortably distended. They cry but this stops when their discomfort passes quite literally with a burp or fart. You can wind them to assist with this but you don't have to hammer the baby's back while you are standing up. Sit down in an upright chair with your baby in your lap, his back to you so that he is facing away from you. Pull him in so that he is right up against your stomach and then rock yourself, and him with you, slowly and gently, forwards and back, for quite a long time (see Figure 14, opposite). A common mistake is to stop too soon. Take a bit longer and the baby eventually burps and settles, if wind was the cause.

A baby will cry if he is hungry, tired, in pain, uncomfortable, angry, frightened or unhappy. He will not cry just to

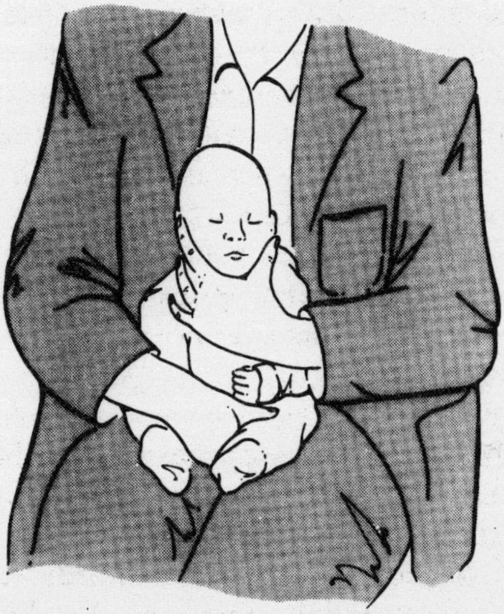

Figure 14 Winding

get his own back on his mother, though it may feel like that. Nor, when tiny, is he likely to learn to cry in order to get his own way. Don't listen to those who say, 'He's putting it on, there are no tears.' It is often the case that genuine crying in the first few weeks of life is unaccompanied by tears. You will not spoil him by picking him up when he cries. Indeed, you may make him more secure. In one study, babies under one year old who were picked up soon after they started crying (not absolutely immediately after every whimper) cried less in their second year of life than those who had earlier been left to cry.

Some babies cry more than others; it is a reflection of their personality (see above). A few are 'screamers' and react with noisy protest to any disturbance of their world.

The interesting thing about such babies is that, whereas they are hell to live with at the time, they usually grow up into normal children. The task for their parents is merely to survive, comfort them and wait for it to pass (informing the neighbours if necessary in order to avoid an unexpected visit from social services).

There is no sound so aversive and intrusive as your own baby crying. It is impossible to ignore and puts you in a series of unpleasant frames of mind: apprehensive, anxious, irritated, exasperated, feeling useless as a mother, and then downright bloody angry. Quite apart from your wish to ease your baby's distress, you experience a powerful feeling of being driven to stop it. This is something evolution has made a present of for you – it obviously helps the survival of the species if mothers are wired up to respond promptly to their offspring's distress. Evolution tends to have it in for mothers.

Grandmothers frequently state that your baby is crying because he is 'overtired'. You may think this is absurd because if the baby was tired he would go to sleep. Nevertheless, the sense of what they are saying is correct, although they are using an unhelpful word. Learning to fall asleep is a skill. What seems to happen is that some babies are slow to pick it up. Although they are tired, they lack the ability to fall asleep. They cannot soothe themselves into a pre-sleep state so cannot get started on the process of falling asleep. They do not know how to close their eyes and float; they have not yet learned to suck their thumb and cannot, therefore, soothe themselves to sleep. They feel uncomfortably tired but can do nothing to resolve it (and you, too, probably know the feeling). This makes them upset and irritable so they find it even more difficult to find the knack of relaxing and letting go in order to fall asleep. Their obvious upset should result in eliciting calming and soothing handling from you but may backfire if they just succeed in exporting their own insomnia to you.

Thumbs or fingers are good for comfort sucking and therefore self-soothing. But when a baby is only a few weeks old he often has difficulty finding his own thumb to suck. He doesn't seem to know where it is or how to get it into his mouth. A dummy (see page 116–17) is an excellent substitute but your baby may have to learn how to use it. You will probably have to put it in his mouth *and* hold it in place for a few minutes to start off with. Although unfashionable, a well-designed dummy offers the baby the chance to use sucking as a self-soothing activity.

Babies will root and suck in any case when they are distressed but don't always find anything satisfying to suck. Some mothers, noticing these attempts to suck assume their baby is hungry and feed him. He sucks for comfort but takes food on board as well so gets uncomfortably distended (and fatter). Discomfort makes him upset and he sucks for comfort, increasing his distension as he does so. A vicious spiral is established.

If the baby is not settling to sleep when you put him down, try wrapping him up tightly by swaddling him in a blanket (see page 106). This provides him with a sense of being contained and restrains his flailing limbs. Some babies, like some adults, twitch as they are falling asleep. This is quite normal but is a nuisance if it makes a baby's arms give such a violent jerk that it wakes him up. He will be startled into confused wakefulness and cry.

EVENING FRETTING

Between about three and twelve weeks of age it is very common indeed for babies to fret, grizzle, whinge or be otherwise unsettled in the evening. This light crying which stops when you pick the baby up and soothe him can follow a perfectly settled day. It is not just the appearance of your husband returning from work which triggers it; it happens at weekends too. Both you and your husband become adept at eating with one hand (baby in the other). In a few weeks' time you may wonder if you will ever again be able to have supper without baby constantly present like Banquo's ghost. Don't panic – it is a temporary stage. Most babies are settling down to sleep before your supper (and remaining there) by three months.

It is possible that your baby is hungry, as the supply of some mothers' breast milk may be relatively low in the evenings though it won't be 'thin' or 'weak' as is sometimes asserted. A hungry baby, however, is unlikely to stop crying for long when you pick him up. Obviously it is sensible to offer a grizzling baby a feed if you think he is hungry, but remember that it is easy to be misled as to the cause of his grizzling. An unsettled baby will suck for comfort rather than hunger. You can get an idea as to whether he is hungry as a result of low milk supply by seeing how long he will sleep before waking for a night feed. However, most babies who grizzle in the evening cannot settle themselves and feel uncomfortable rather than hungry.

The need to learn self-soothing techniques, which we discussed in the previous section, is a reason why evening fretting is such a common problem. This is the time when everyone wants the baby to go to sleep. He may or may not be tired, but either way cannot get himself to sleep. After a bit his parents think it's actually that he won't (rather than can't) and it seems to them like a battle of wills. They get ratty and this unsettles him further. The fretting is thus a combination of his inability to settle himself and his response to your (understandable) impatience.

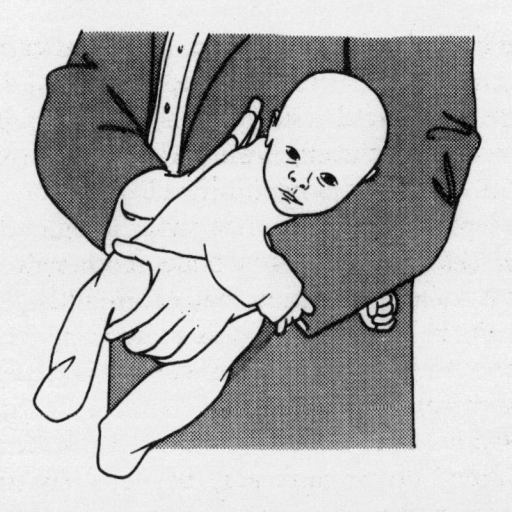

Figure 15 Carrying a baby along the forearm

The answer for most fretting babies is to go with it and not keep trying to settle them in their crib or cot. Pick them up, and if they don't settle immediately, place them along your forearm as shown above and pace (walk slowly up and down your hall or around your sitting room). The rhythm of steady walking provides a regular jiggle of about one 'bouncelet' per second which is inherently soothing. Your free hand can hold his dummy in place. This method is better for your back than using an over-the-shoulder carrying technique because you are less likely to slop into a pregnancy posture with resultant backache.

Your basic task is to be there for your baby and continue your efforts to soothe him, not to find the elusive remedy for his crying. If it is the case (as is sometimes said) that anxious mothers communicate their anxiety to their babies then it is probably because they become too impatient to do anything soothing for long enough. If they anxiously keep trying different tactics – give him a feed, try to wind him, put him down, pick him up, bounce him, sing to him, etc. – but nothing is carried out for long enough then he will get irritable or anxious, not being satisfied by any manoeuvre and not knowing what is coming next.

This is one explanation as to why grandmothers can sometimes settle a baby when his mother can't. They achieve this merely by sitting and rocking him for longer than the mother has had the patience or confidence to do. Mothers tend to be too anxious or impatient to persist with soothing because they have other things to do and are worried that they are not doing the right thing anyway (or even 'letting him get away with it', 'spoiling him', etc., etc.). It is always much easier if it isn't your baby. Get the issue of responsibility straight: your first duty is to survive – to be with your baby and try to comfort him. It is asking too much of yourself to solve the problem of his unhappiness all the time. No parent, whatever the age of their child, has the responsibility to ensure their child's continual happiness. It just cannot be done.

A further reason for other people being able to settle your baby more easily than you can is because the baby may smell your milk. He may become distracted by this, even if he is not actually hungry, because the smell of milk reminds him of comfortable feelings yet these are not what he is experiencing.

A tiny baby crying at night who does not settle after a feed and subsequent prolonged attempts to wind him can be taken into bed with you without any fear that this will lead to a bad habit being established. You will doubtless hear all sorts of tuttings and warnings to the effect that you are making a rod for your own back, etc. Quite frankly, after an hour's pacing, you will probably welcome a rod for your back; it would come in useful just to keep you upright.

But there is a more serious point. Babies do not learn that quickly – if they did, life would be a lot easier. Taking your baby into bed with you when he does not settle after a feed or after waking at night will not set up an inevitable bad habit. More importantly, if it means you (and he) can get some sleep that you would not otherwise have had, you won't get on each other's nerves so much the following day. You will have more opportunity to enjoy each other, which is by far the more important issue.

CRYING WHICH WILL NOT STOP

Forceful crying which persists in spite of your best attempts to comfort your baby needs more active management. Crying throughout the day is likely to be caused by hunger or pain. Persistent crying in the evenings which does not respond to straightforward measures (such as picking him up, winding, trying a dummy, trying a feed, and pacing) will probably be colic.

The first thing to do with the problem of crying throughout the day is to check your baby's weight gain. A thriving baby who is eating well and putting on about a pound (450 grams) a fortnight is unlikely to be continually hungry. If he is underweight, then he is probably persistently hungry because his daily intake of milk is too low and the remedy is obvious: offer him longer at each feed and introduce an extra feed or two. Don't worry about routines yet. Indeed, a common cause for low nutritional intake is a parent's (or maternity nurse's) premature enthusiasm for feeding routines with a breast-fed baby.

Alternatively, you may simply not have realised that his total daily intake of milk is low because you are pleased that he has a good appetite. In other words he may be starting each feed well but his feeding may be too greedy and disrupted by wind or he may be losing some of what he eats by throwing it up later (paradoxically, throwing up immediately after a feed may be the result of over-feeding). Very few babies have trouble absorbing enough nutrition from ordinary formula milks. Occasionally, though most unusually, your baby may be failing to gain weight because of some more complex problem. Discuss the matter with your health visitor or with your doctor.

A baby who has previously been relatively uncomplaining but then starts to cry throughout the day (and night) may well be in pain from an invisible cause. The most likely candidate is a middle ear infection for which he will probably need antibiotics. This means taking him to the doctor to have his ear drums examined. If he has got a roaring middle ear infection he will also have a raised temperature and may well throw up, too, which can confuse you as to the source of the pain.

A small number of babies (perhaps one in 20) will develop colic at about the third week of their lives. This produces explosive outbursts of crying every evening which is more severe, protracted and unresponsive to soothing than evening fretting. When severe, the baby draws his knees up on to his chest and gives every impression of being racked by spasms of tummy pain. Matters only subside after several hours. The whole problem disappears magically at ten to fourteen weeks (which is why it is called three-month colic).

A considerable amount of nonsense has been written about colic. Some professionals who should know better deny its existence and don't seem to have enough experience to tell the difference between colic and evening fretting (and certainly many people use the term 'colic' as a descriptive term for any evening crying). Others say that it is caused by maternal anxiety communicated to the child. Many mothers with colicky babies are indeed anxious but this is more likely to be effect rather than cause. More recently, a view has been expressed that colic is 'developmental', in other words that all babies do it at this age (yet they don't).

One problem is that no one has ever demonstrated the underlying cause of colic. It looks to an observer like the sort of pain produced by spasm of part of the intestines and a number of affected babies are helped by medicines which relieve gut spasm (Infacol, etc.). However, these are not helpful in all cases.

Perhaps because of this, a number of theories abound and this is another area in which you will hear conflicting advice from all quarters rather than sympathy which would be more to the point. Once again, everyone is an expert when it comes to the persistently crying baby. It is party-time for mother-blamers. Yet if anyone really knew the answer, they would be rich beyond their dreams. A favourite suggestion is that it is something that a breast-feeding mother has been eating – dairy products and salad (of all things) often seem to be blamed. Although a few new babies have persistent discomfort if their mothers eat a *great deal* of garlic or highly spiced foods, or a *great deal* of citrus fruit, we have never ever seen a convincing case of three-month evening colic result from a dietary cause. As the colic is confined to the evenings it is rather hard to see why the baby should only be intolerant of the dietary irritant then. As with any time-limited condition, a large number of treatments for colic (cranial osteopathy, baby massage, etc.) appear to 'work' at about ten to fourteen weeks of age (!).

You may well be told that the problem is wind. It is unlikely that winding will provide more than momentary relief in the case of good-going colic but it is usually impossible to resist the temptation to do it. Attempt it by all means but restrain your (or your husband's) enthusiasm for a result before it takes on the character of a personal challenge.

For severe evening colic, ask your doctor if there is any medicine that he would recommend for your baby. There is no single one which works for all colicky babies but dimethicone (Infacol) drops, which prevent stomach contents foaming, or Gaviscon liquid, which forms a barrier against stomach acid, are sometimes helpful. What often happens is some improvement but not the total abolition which you are hoping for. Unfortunately, dicyclomine (Merbentyl), which was brilliant, is no longer recommended for tiny babies because of a possible link with sudden collapse in a very few cases.

There may not be a suitable or effective medicine for your baby, in which case the task for you is to survive until the baby grows out of it by fourteen weeks at the latest. Mark when this will be on a calendar and cross off each day that passes. That way it won't seem so endless. You will have to comfort your baby each evening for several hours. The situation is truly ghastly. You may not be able to relieve his discomfort much but at least it does him no lasting harm physically or psychologically.

Do not blame yourself if your baby has colic. It does seem to run in some families but is not caused by any aspect of your diet or your state of mind. Share the burden with your husband; recruit some practical help from your mother or his mother. If you can agree a rota, this spares a few arguments about whose turn it is. Do whatever seems best to you. Pace with your baby over your arm, holding a dummy in position with your other hand (plug yourself into a Walkman), wheel him up and down in the pram (inside or outside), take him for evening drives in the car, or rock him in a cradle. Gentle rhythmic movements with a frequency of about one per second are often soothing though he may not actually fall asleep. Try gripe water if you wish but it is not usually very useful. At about eleven weeks you may feel ready to crack. Grit your teeth and see it through. It is not your fault, not the baby's, not your husband's(!), and it will very soon be over.

You will sometimes feel desperate and you may often feel furious with your baby. Such feelings are common. Do share them with someone, preferably a friend who has had a crying baby, your mother or your husband. If you cannot, because no one is there at the time, a telephone service for desperate mothers with crying babies provides a helpline (CRY-SIS: 0171 404 5011). Otherwise, if you feel about to lose your temper, put your baby down gently in his crib or pram and walk into another room for a few minutes. Put some distance between the two of you so you can't lose your self-control and harm him. Shaking or squeezing a baby in anger is terribly dangerous.

FEEDING

Most breast fed babies will still be needing six feeds a day. Very few will maintain a good weight gain with five, and some will need seven. Mothers who are breast feeding may be fortunate and notice a pattern emerging. There might be a general impression of three- to four-hourly feeds during the day, chaotic feeding throughout the evening and the occasional unbroken spell of five hours during the night. It is, however, quite normal for babies to show no sign of any such pattern. Be patient – it is still too early to impose routines. A bottle fed baby may well be thriving on five feeds.

Check your baby's weight to ensure that his growth rate is steady at an average of an ounce a day measured over several days. Don't buy scales for weighing him daily at home; take him to your local clinic once a fortnight. If your health visitor has doubts about his rate of weight gain or if he isn't settling after a feed she will want to see him more frequently. It is important to lay down a secure foundation of adequate milk intake before attempting to introduce a feeding routine at roughly six weeks. You can't impose a routine until you know your baby is putting on the right amount of weight. Beware of getting carried away and fattening him up excessively, though.

If you are breast feeding, start getting your baby used to an occasional bottle during the day so that he adds the skill of teat sucking to his competence at nipple sucking. Knowing that your baby is able to take a bottle is a very useful move which extends beyond the possible night-time advantages of eventually allowing your husband to bale you out in the wee small hours. If your baby will only take from the breast, your mobility during the day will be severely constrained, something which does not matter now, but is likely to be important in a few months' time – even if you are not planning to return to work.

Put in the bottle almost anything civilised and safe: expressed milk, camomile tea, baby fruit juice from the chemist, even previously boiled or bottled water (Evian, Volvic, Highland Spring or Sainsbury's Natural Scottish Spring have the correct electrolyte balance) if he will take it. Remember that breast-fed babies are used to taking their milk at a constant body temperature (quite warm) which means you may have better success with whatever is in the bottle if it is slightly warmer than you would like to drink it yourself. Although most mothers would rather not introduce sweetened drinks, sometimes it is the only way of coaxing a breast-hooked baby to take from a bottle. Breast milk is actually quite sweet – it is common for breast-fed babies to appear horrified when they taste water.

The point is to get him used to taking a teat every day, not to provide nutrition but to get him used to sucking on a teat rather than a nipple. If he has been using a dummy you will probably find he takes to a bottle more easily.

Incidentally, you may notice that you are continually hungry and crave sweet things. Although you may be anxious to recover your precious figure, now is not the time to lose weight. Listen to your body and eat what you like so long as you maintain a reasonably balanced diet. You don't need a special diet if you're lactating but you do need to eat more than usual.

MASTITIS

If you are unlucky enough to get mastitis, the most likely time for it is between three and five weeks after the birth. The first thing you might be aware of is feeling slightly 'fluey'. You may then notice a hard lump in one of your breasts, slightly tender at first, then becoming very tender, red, painful and throbbing over the next few days. By this time you will be feeling quite ill in yourself and have a temperature.

What has almost certainly happened is that a milk duct inside your breast has become blocked. Milk builds up behind the blockage and, as the back-pressure increases, it seeps out into the tissues around the duct. This causes tenderness and a local inflammatory reaction. It creates a fertile breeding ground for bacteria and a raging infection very commonly develops. This is what makes you feel ill with flu-like aches and weakness, though if you are very sleep-deprived and already feeling like death, you may not notice these symptoms very much. Bacteria can enter breast tissue from the bloodstream or even through a badly cracked nipple. If unchecked, a bacterial infection can lead to a breast abscess which is more serious and will probably need admission to hospital – so this needs to be avoided by prompt treatment.

Matters hinge upon whether you have a temperature so take it in order to check. If you have got one it means that you may well have a bacterial infection so *contact your GP immediately* (it is always Friday evening when these things happen). He or she will need to establish whether infection really is present. If so, he or she will prescribe a course of antibiotics to kill the bacteria and prevent an abscess forming. Get these from the chemist and down your throat *as soon as possible*. They work within 48 hours so if the lump and your temperature have not begun to subside by this time contact your doctor again. You should continue to feed. Contrary to popular belief, neither the antibiotics nor the infection will harm the baby and his feeding will keep the breast drained. Only if your doctor tells you that you have an actual abscess will you need to stop feeding.

If you catch the blockage before bacterial infection has set in, you will not have a temperature. Don't squeeze the lump because that will force more milk out into the surrounding breast tissue. You may be able to unblock the duct by turning your baby round to face the other way for a feed (his legs under your arm rather than resting on your lap). This is called the 'football' hold, which alters the pattern of suction on the nipple ducts. Then while he is sucking, stroke downwards over the lump with your fingers or an Afro comb. Take a hot bath and carry out the same stroking action, alternating it with a hot flannel applied to the affected breast. Over the next few days, keep

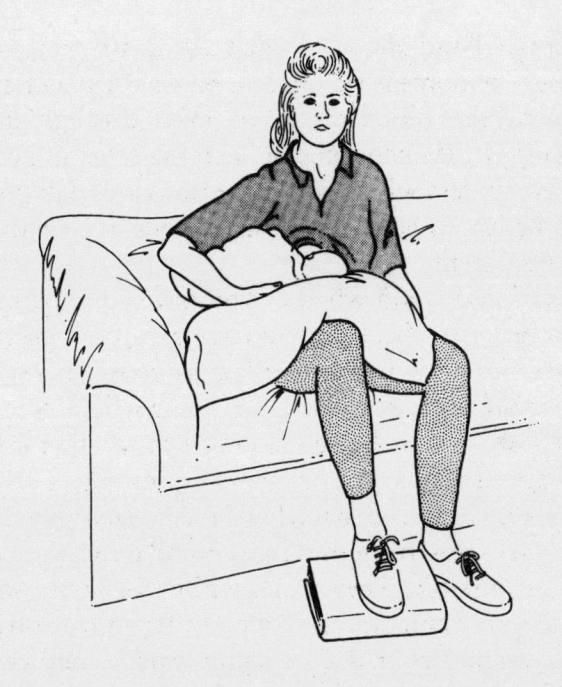

Figure 16 The 'football' hold

taking your temperature in order to detect any infection at the earliest possible stage. Bear in mind that mastitis may recur; some women are unlucky enough to have ducts that keep blocking.

STAGE 5

Nudging back into the fast lane

16

Six weeks onwards: nudging back into the fast lane

By six weeks your mother will have departed and if you had a maternity nurse, she will have moved on. You find yourself left quite literally holding the baby. You will probably gulp a little as your self-confidence wobbles. Evenings may still be tricky and hurdles like the returns to sex and work loom ominously. The family show must be kept on the road and you need to continue with good-enough parenting. Yet you will be nudging towards normality and feeling more at ease with yourself as a mother. Your baby will start to smile broadly and the emotional impact on you will be wonderful.

SIX-WEEK CHECK

At six weeks after the birth, you will have a physical check-up. This is not an indication that you should now be back to normal as you won't be and won't feel you are. In fact, you are quite likely to feel sleep-deprived and will welcome your now well-established habit of the afternoon rest.

The check-up is a straightforward process and can be undertaken by your GP or your obstetrician, but you should be prepared for an internal examination. The purpose of this exercise is to ensure that your uterus is shrinking down and in the right place, that your cervix is satisfactory, that you are not still bleeding and your stitches have healed. At the end of the examination you will be asked about contraception.

SEX

Until they have had a reassurance that all is anatomically present and correct down below, most women feel very nervous about resuming sexual activity. Even when the six-week check has given them a confirmation that sex is mechanically possible, the vast majority will find themselves devoid of any libido whatsoever. This poses quite a problem since their husbands may be consumed with lust. If your stitches are fully healed, and the vast majority will be, the only sensible thing to do is buy some Senselle lubricant or KY jelly, apply liberally and get on with it (practising your pelvic floor exercises at the same time). Rest assured that nobody has a scintillating sex life and a new baby at the same time. It might be worth considering why not.

Most women are simply very tired indeed after six weeks of broken nights and chronic sleep deprivation is no aphrodisiac. Many do not feel sexually attractive in themselves, particularly if they are lactating. A common experience of women with new babies is that their breasts leak in an off-putting fashion during sex (especially so if they

16

Six weeks onwards: nudging back into the fast lane

By six weeks your mother will have departed and if you had a maternity nurse, she will have moved on. You find yourself left quite literally holding the baby. You will probably gulp a little as your self-confidence wobbles. Evenings may still be tricky and hurdles like the returns to sex and work loom ominously. The family show must be kept on the road and you need to continue with good-enough parenting. Yet you will be nudging towards normality and feeling more at ease with yourself as a mother. Your baby will start to smile broadly and the emotional impact on you will be wonderful.

SIX-WEEK CHECK

At six weeks after the birth, you will have a physical check-up. This is not an indication that you should now be back to normal as you won't be and won't feel you are. In fact, you are quite likely to feel sleep-deprived and will welcome your now well-established habit of the afternoon rest.

The check-up is a straightforward process and can be undertaken by your GP or your obstetrician, but you should be prepared for an internal examination. The purpose of this exercise is to ensure that your uterus is shrinking down and in the right place, that your cervix is satisfactory, that you are not still bleeding and your stitches have healed. At the end of the examination you will be asked about contraception.

SEX

Until they have had a reassurance that all is anatomically present and correct down below, most women feel very nervous about resuming sexual activity. Even when the six-week check has given them a confirmation that sex is mechanically possible, the vast majority will find themselves devoid of any libido whatsoever. This poses quite a problem since their husbands may be consumed with lust. If your stitches are fully healed, and the vast majority will be, the only sensible thing to do is buy some Senselle lubricant or KY jelly, apply liberally and get on with it (practising your pelvic floor exercises at the same time). Rest assured that nobody has a scintillating sex life and a new baby at the same time. It might be worth considering why not.

Most women are simply very tired indeed after six weeks of broken nights and chronic sleep deprivation is no aphrodisiac. Many do not feel sexually attractive in themselves, particularly if they are lactating. A common experience of women with new babies is that their breasts leak in an off-putting fashion during sex (especially so if they experience one of those rarities of the postnatal period – an orgasm). There is also always the risk that the baby will start to cry while you are ensconced (they always seem to know exactly when one of you is approaching *il momento supremo*). Perhaps most insidiously of all, the sexual demands of the husband come across just like that – more demands. At a time when the baby is making substantial claims on her time and energy, the thought of having to accommodate another person who is insisting upon physical contact is sometimes too much for the woman.

MAINTAINING YOUR RELATIONSHIP WITH YOUR HUSBAND

For most young families, the early months after the first few postnatal days are quite a strain. At the heart of this is the problem of three people learning to live together as a family where previously there were only two. It is hard enough for two people to learn to live together as a couple (remember all those rows!). Now the task is more complicated. One of the reasons for this is that not only is there a third person in the family but the family roles of the adults have doubled up: each is now not only a wife or husband but a parent too. It is not always clear which role takes priority. The problem over sex is a common flashpoint for a row about this competition for role priorities ('You spend all your time worrying about the baby; I need some of you too') especially as it becomes clear, as it will when the baby starts to cry during foreplay, that the mother role trumps the wife role when small babies are concerned.

Learning to live as a three-person, two-generation household is not easy and involves some discomfort. It is particularly difficult when you, as the mother/wife (and, yes, the cook, cleaner, shopper, telephone answering service, daughter, daughter-in-law, person-wanted-back-at-the-office, etc.) are beginning to feel increasingly tired and slow as you find yourself entirely surrounded by baby. It comes especially sharply into focus if your baby is a prickly, dissatisfied individual rather than one possessing an easy-going, sunny disposition.

There are some things which you can do to ease the situation. In essence, many of these mean taking the trouble to look after yourself. If you can do this, you will feel less drained, more resourceful and therefore not so resentful at having to devote some of your time to your husband. This means that he, in turn, will not feel so crabby at having to run rings round you in order to support your mothering. If you feel that life is on your side, you can afford to be generous-minded and this brings back dividends in any relationship.

There is a general risk that, because of the demands of your baby, your own sources of stimulation which kept you an interesting person in the past will wither because you can't get to them. You won't want to leave your baby to get out to the cinema or theatre, and going out to dinner parties seems like an awe-inspiring organisational challenge. (In any case, will you be able to stay awake until the pudding?) It may, in fact, be easier to have a friend or two over to an unceremonious supper than go out, if only because you can control the timetable.

The odds are that your state of mind is not suited to reading the Booker prize short-list in between feeds, but you may be able to read a newspaper. Keep your brain ticking over so that you have something to talk about apart from your delivery. If there is a way in which you can manage to have something to look forward to each day (a friend dropping over, buying *yourself* a new tracksuit), you will stave off the comfortable, though suffocating, monotony that it is otherwise so easy to sink into.

It is not always easy to keep a focus on your husband. It may seem to you that he is a grown-up and well able to look after himself. Yet plenty of women feel guilty in the evening when they realise they have been too distracted and busy to prepare a meal for their husband who comes in tired after a day's work, or find themselves unable to discover any interest whatsoever in his activities when he describes them. This sort of thing tends to become intensified when each party tries to coerce the other into a one-down position, often along the lines of, 'I've had a dreadful day; you should have been able to tell; you would have been able to tell if you'd paid me any attention; it's all your fault I'm upset; now it's up to you to make me feel better', etc., etc. The adult way of managing such conflict is to spot it coming and ward it off.

Lay in a supply of instant meals to compensate for any failure on your part to prepare supper, tell your other half straightforwardly how you are feeling (but without playing excessively for sympathy), and ask them to do something specific which will help you (such as walk the baby for a bit). In very general terms, being open and explicit about how you are feeling is better than playing the game of waiting for the other person to guess, and building up smouldering resentment when they seem to be slow on the uptake.

The whole problem of attending to your husband is compounded by the fact that most babies between the ages of three and ten weeks are at their worst in the evening, or just at the time that husbands return home. Most babies tend to be unsettled between the hours of 6 p.m. and 10 p.m. and may indeed be crying continually. Some babies will even have colic. This means that parents cannot even sit down together for supper in peace. There is no magic answer to all this and the period from three weeks to three months after birth is a difficult patch for everyone. It helps if both parents realise that a parent's first duty is to survive, so that they grit their teeth and get on with it. It is a strain on individuals and on marriages but it gets better, it really does.

MAINTAINING YOUR SOCIAL NETWORK

Women with new babies can become lonely, perhaps for the first time in their lives. They can also, believe it or not, feel slightly bored. Accordingly, you may find it wise to nurture your social network by keeping links with your friends. See friends for coffee mornings, go to postnatal classes, use the telephone. Ring up the other people in your antenatal class and send out birth notification cards with small handwritten notes on them to other people you would like to see. Social isolation can creep up on you if you become too obsessed by babycare, and social contacts are one source of stimulation which can be lost without you noticing.

Friends enable you to do things for yourself. For instance, you can go swimming with a friend who also has a baby about the same age. She looks after the babies while you do a couple of lengths and you can then do the same. Likewise, if you go shopping, she can mind the babies and utter judgements as you try on various garments. Keep yourself in focus.

FATIGUE

Tiny babies are tiring. A common pattern is for new mothers to throw themselves into babycare, allowing only the baby's wants and needs to dominate their minds, and hitting a trough of exhaustion at ten weeks after the birth. It may creep up on them unawares because they allow their standards to drift. A night in which they are only woken once for a feed becomes a 'really good night', even if the total sleep time is six and a half hours in two stages.

Firstly, you must still try to get some sleep during the day, even if you feel you don't really need it. If you are unable to sleep, practise the relaxation techniques taught at your antenatal classes or buy a relaxation tape. Most babies do not sleep through the night until they are about three months old – in spite of what their mothers might tell you – and therefore your sleep deprivation will continue to accumulate. If your baby seems to make it impossible for you to sleep during the day, it might be worth asking your mother, mother-in-law or even a good friend to take him for a walk two or three afternoons a week.

While you need to keep your social life actively ticking over, avoid late dinner parties, *never go out two nights running* and be careful of long drives to see the baby's grandparents.

At the same time, think what tasks can be delegated: walking up and down with a fretting baby is one. Don't feel that you ought to do everything for your baby. Even breast feeding needs to be considered in this light. If you are desperately tired at ten weeks (especially if you are back at work) and have satisfactorily established breast feeding, consider the advantages of combining breast during the day with a bottle at night. This will enable you and your husband to share the joy of night feeds. Obviously only a few babies are going to adapt to a bottle just like that (those that used a dummy in the early stages will do so more readily) and it is sensible to try to get them used to a bottle during daylight hours first. The hazards of mixing breast and bottle in the early weeks before your milk is established do not apply at this stage. You can, of course, put your own expressed breast milk in the bottle if you want to, or if you are uneasy as to whether formula milk is good enough (actually it is).

If you and your husband are going to share any task which involves getting up at night, the best advice is to have a system of alternating nights on duty; an alternating one-in-two on call rota. This avoids the business of each partner waking but pretending to be asleep when the baby cries, waiting for the other one to go and soothe him. Such waiting can go on for a long time as bluff is called or before negotiations start ('I've had a hard day at the office' versus 'I'm exhausted having looked after him all day') and eventually angry recriminations result, so that in the end two adults have lost the same amount of sleep unnecessarily. It is easier for both to know what their responsibilities are beforehand.

Use weekends to catch up on the week. If you have a nanny and can afford it, ask her to stay on for Saturday morning to give you a chance to lie in. There's no need to feel guilty about this. Remember that it is the quality of your time with your baby that counts, not the sheer quantity. Your husband needs to spend some time with his baby too – he can take the baby out in the afternoon so you can get your usual siesta.

DEPRESSION

At about ten weeks, given that the chances are that you will be feeling supremely exhausted and possibly demoralised, how can you tell whether you have got postnatal depression? The latter is not rare – though the severe form of mental disorder known variously as postpartum psychosis or puerperal psychosis is extremely rare (and so we are not covering it in this book). Most studies suggest that, across the board, about one woman in ten will experience some form of depression. It is probable that the sort of anticipatory planning and coping which we are talking about in this book will minimise the likelihood of its occurrence.

Depression is more than feeling fed up or demoralised. It is a morbidly unhappy state which affects adversely all the positive things in one's mind: the capacity to enjoy things, to look forward to events, to accommodate minor mishaps, to be realistic about one's shortcomings, to feel some self-confidence and to summon up sufficient energy. If someone is depressed, they will usually experience irrational and unjustifiable guilt, anger and anxiety, they will be tired but unable to sleep, and find themselves beset by painful doubts and memories.

They are quite likely to come across to others as ratty and irritable with worries that are hard for others to take seriously – not all women who are depressed are predominantly tearful and miserable. It is also the case that they will feel tired and lose their libido but these particular findings are not very helpful indicators of depression in the first few months of new motherhood when fatigue and a lack of interest in sex are virtually universal.

What are the key danger signals? Firstly that there is an obvious change of mood so that you find yourself repeatedly snapping at everybody or bursting into tears in a way that just isn't you. Secondly, and coupled with this, there are four typical patterns of thought and feelings, any of which are likely to be recognised in yourself or by your husband. All these are exaggerations of occasional thoughts and feelings that just about everyone gets.

- *Persistently* thinking that the baby is a mistake and that you have married the wrong husband. Everyone has such thoughts sometimes (particularly at about eight weeks after childbirth) but in this instance you find you cannot rid yourself of them.
- *Serious* loss of confidence so that you feel *persistently* inadequate, incompetent and useless as a mother and wife.
- *Dreadful* anxiety about your baby coupled with a sense of imminent disaster or a conviction that there is something horribly wrong with him that you haven't been told about.
- Finding yourself getting *repeatedly* angry with your baby, even hating him, perhaps to the extent that you have to cover this up with an exaggerated public display of affection.

If you think any or all of these apply to you, the first thing is to talk about it with your husband, friend or health visitor. This is not easy because one of the perverse feelings which is part of depression is a sense of shame and a belief that in some way it is your fault and you ought to be able to pull yourself together without outside help, even though this is patently impossible.

Sometimes putting everything into words is enough to reverse the process but if not, *you must consult your GP*. Take your husband along with you. Once again, the act of explaining how you feel to someone who is prepared to listen may prove sufficient help in its own right, especially if you come to realise that becoming depressed at this time is in no way your fault and does not betray a previously unsuspected flaw in your personality. If talking about how you feel is not enough, there are various treatments which can be employed.

Probably the most widely used are antidepressant drugs. These act to relieve depression; they are not tranquillisers (though some may make you drowsy). The important thing is to keep taking them for as long as you are advised to – don't stop as soon as you cheer up since you may find yourself slipping back down again. They often take a couple of weeks and sometimes a month to have the desired effect; don't expect an instant cure. Stick to the dose prescribed. You may need to take them for several months but you needn't worry about getting addicted to them. Most antidepressant drugs are compatible with breast feeding but make a point of discussing this with your GP.

Some doctors believe that it is sensible to prescribe the hormone progesterone which is produced by the body at a high level during pregnancy and falls gradually afterwards. By replacing this, some of the mood changes which occur in the postnatal weeks may be offset. It is not well absorbed if taken as an ordinary pill so it is usually given as suppositories.

A newer treatment for depression is to discuss your thoughts with a therapist who helps you to question some of the assumptions and beliefs you have been making in your thinking. This is called cognitive therapy and is mainly practised in hospital clinics rather than in general practice. It is not very likely that the sort of psychotherapy which concentrates on your own early relationships is going to be helpful at this stage.

Whichever approach is taken in your case, the general

advice is to see it through. But if you find yourself getting worse in spite of treatment then you must tell your doctor. The problem is that partial treatment is likely to lead to a relapse. If postnatal depression goes untreated or only partly treated it can persist for a long time and cause considerable misery. By definition you cannot snap out of it using willpower alone. Don't believe the people who imply you can.

GOOD HABITS

At six weeks you can begin to shift the balance of power. Hitherto you have been running very much on your baby's timetable, responsive to his needs at the time they arise. You can now try, gently and gradually, to move these feeding and sleeping requirements into a more predictable pattern. This will enable you to keep yourself in focus.

FEEDING

As far as feeding goes, bottle-fed babies will by now be on a reasonably predictable four-hour routine. Many breast-fed babies will also have organised themselves into a loose four-hourly pattern, having five to six feeds during a 24-hour period. Other breast-fed babies will be hopelessly unpredictable or, worse still, continue to want feeding every two hours. These latter babies are usually taking the same amount of milk over 24 hours (so you are producing the required amount) but they are taking smaller amounts more frequently.

Provided that your baby's weight gain is satisfactory, now is the time you can start the business of establishing a feeding routine – if, of course, you want to. Just watch out for the possibility that your baby is going through a minor greedy patch (as a result of a growth spurt) when he demands (and needs) more milk. This is something which tends to happen for a few days at about five to six weeks and again at nine to ten weeks. You will know when it happens because your breasts will be less full than usual and your baby will not settle after a feed. Avoid introducing a routine at this point – feed your baby more frequently and your breasts will get the message that they need to produce more milk. This will take two to three days.

Otherwise, over the next week or so, aim to lengthen gradually the time between his feeds. Find two days that are reasonably clear of commitments. Perhaps start by setting a minimum of three hours between feeds during the day – forget the evenings and nights for the time being. If your baby starts to agitate at two and a half hours after the last feed, don't opt for the easy solution of putting him to the breast but work away with distraction techniques – jiggling him, taking him for a walk or car ride or even giving him a bath. Keep stringing him out to a minimum of three hours between successive daytime feeds.

Once he is comfortably established on a three-hour minimum interval during the day for at least three continuous days, you can move to setting the minimum at three and a quarter hours between feeds. Once he has settled on that for three days, move to three and a half hours between feeds and so on until there is roughly a four-hour interval. You can afford to be flexible about the timing of early evening feeds. If he has colic in the evenings, wait until this subsides at about twelve weeks before trying to fiddle with evening feed timings.

DAYTIME SLEEPS

If you make a point of ensuring that your baby is put down lying flat for his daytime sleeps (as opposed to sitting slumped in the car seat), you have a better chance of avoiding the catnap syndrome of brief, unsustained spells of sleep. This is the situation in which he naps for brief periods during the day, dozing off in the car seat for five minutes, and is then woken as you sweep him indoors and whisk his hat off, putting him in a bouncing chair while you gas on the phone. He dozes again, subsequently being jolted awake by you scooping him up to take him upstairs for his afternoon nap (while you have yours), whereupon he doesn't (and neither do you). He never gets the chance to get into a good habit of sustained sleep.

Help your baby to learn how to settle himself to sleep during the day. On the whole, a baby will find it easier to sleep through the night when he has learnt how to fall asleep on his own during the day. Put him down for a good rest at least once during the day – early afternoon or late morning (or both). Jiggle the crib/cot/pram but don't pace up and down with him because he will come to think that he is only able to fall asleep in your arms. Help him to learn how to settle himself. You can let him cry a bit at such times so long as he doesn't get too steamed up. Just keep gently and gradually nudging him to do what you want him to do.

Once again, go more slowly with colicky babies. Because they inevitably spend every evening being paced until they settle, they have less opportunity to learn how to fall asleep alone. There's nothing you should do about this beyond trying to create that opportunity during the day when settling them for a nap. Don't try to give up pacing in the evenings. The colic will have settled by fourteen weeks and you can sort things out once it has done so.

Avoid out-and-out confrontations and show-downs because these don't help him learn new skills. You might think it necessary or helpful to demonstrate to him that you are in charge but it won't actually make any difference at this age. He won't learn that he is less powerful than you because his conceptualisation of personal relationships has not developed to allow that level of sophistication. He is still at the stage of a basic assumption that the world revolves around him and a single demonstration that it does not will not change his mind or force the pace of his conceptual development; he can't yet think like that. Forget, therefore, about trying to show him who's boss at this stage – you might become so exhausted by a fight to the finish that you wonder whether you really are in charge.

HELPING YOUR BABY TO SLEEP THROUGH THE NIGHT (!)

Small babies sleep for more hours in the day than adults but they have not yet learned the cues which induce sleep at night rather than in the day. For the first few weeks after birth they tend to sleep on an eight-hour cycle, only slowly shifting towards a pattern of one major sleep burst and one or two shorter ones. If you allow your baby to sleep for too long during the day you may find that he is shifting his major sleep session into daylight hours with interesting periods of alert sociability in the small hours of the morning.

For such reasons it is wise to wake him after four hours' sleep for any *daytime* nap – and for the same reason *not* to wake him during the night. Most mothers find that they have more success with night feeds (or the lack of them) if they allow the baby to wake spontaneously for them.

Most babies start to sleep through the night (a decent stretch of eight to twelve hours) at around three months. Provided he is having enough milk during the day, between the age of seven and ten weeks, with any luck, he will manage to sleep for a five- or six-hour stretch. The problem might be that you find it is the 'wrong' six-hour stretch (e.g. between 8 p.m. and 2 a.m.) and wonder whether to wake him for a feed before you go to bed. Although the temptation to wake him up at 11 o'clock to get a feed in before you crash out is hard to resist, what seems to happen is that, having been woken, he is sleepy (!) and therefore does not feed as well as he would have had he woken on his own. So he still wakes for a feed later during the night.

His sleeping time *will lengthen* over the next few weeks. If you keep waking him up in the night you may well miss this magical milestone because you won't be giving him the opportunity to demonstrate his ability to go for a longer period between his night-time feeds. If you allow him to wake spontaneously, what you will probably find is that he naturally lengthens the interval between feeds; he is doing it himself.

There is a helpful interplay between the development of longer sleep–wake cycles and longer feed–hunger cycles. Waking him for a night feed interferes with this and will make it more difficult for him to adjust to longer periods between night feeds which is the necessary preparation before dropping a night feed altogether. Babies don't suddenly sleep for eight hours, they gradually lengthen the time they are content to go without food. Therefore, before he gives up demanding a night feed, you are likely to have a few unsatisfactory nights when he wakes at a worse time than usual – say at 5 a.m. rather than at 3 a.m. Although this is pretty exhausting for you, remember that it will not be for ever and is actually a step in the right direction. In the throes of struggling with a baby who just will not sleep at night, you may be tempted to introduce solid food 'to fill him up'. There is no point in doing any of this before twelve weeks unless you are professionally advised to do so.

As it happens, all babies wake during the night, but only some cry. These are the ones who are noticed; they make sure of that. Unless your baby is hungry, the problem is not, therefore, so much that he wakes, rather that he cannot get himself back off to sleep. He has not yet learned how to settle back to sleep on his own and cries for his mother to make a nipple or teat available for him to soothe himself on. (See daytime sleeps on page 174–5).

If you are fortunate enough to have a baby who sleeps for a twelve-hour stretch at night, remember that it will be impossible to fit in five feeds at four-hour intervals during the day. You may have to reduce the four-hour interval between feeds, rather than dropping a feed as most babies are happier on five feeds a day at this stage.

TALKING TO YOUR BABY

Babies love to be talked to and respond to it with increasing excitement as they get older. Talking to your baby helps his development as well as being fun in its own right. In the first place it helps build his language development, even before he can understand the words you use. He learns to associate your varying facial expressions with the different sounds of your voice. He learns the rhythms and sounds of the language you use.

Most importantly, he learns the art of turn-taking. This probably started even earlier when you began to feed him. Babies suck in bursts so he would suck for a bit and then stop. You would jiggle the nipple in his mouth and he would get going again. Without thinking about it, you and he established a pattern of give-and-take. This is fundamental for learning how to talk with other people – speaking and listening in turn. It is an experience which carries on through the way you talk to him even before he can reply. You find that you and he begin to mesh. You do something and he, in turn, responds. Or, indeed, the other way around. He does something and watches you respond. And then he responds to your response.

One of the most obvious things about adults and babies is the extent to which adults imitate babies (rather than vice versa which is what everyone thinks). This is very obvious when babies start to talk but actually starts even before they begin to babble. Adults, especially mothers, imitate their baby's facial expressions. By doing so they reflect the baby's feelings back to him. The mother's face, already the most fascinating thing in his visual world, becomes a mirror for the baby. He sees his feelings copied in her face. In fact, if the mother keeps a still, unresponsive face her baby becomes distressed.

At about six weeks, babies develop an infectious social smile. They begin to smile radiantly when someone looks at them face-to-face. It is a real social encounter. People will say to you 'Have you got a smile out of him yet?' But it is more than that. If he smiles at you, you will smile back. You will imitate him. In fact, you don't have to smile at him to get a smile but he will get one out of you all right. At first, a baby only needs to see a pair of eyes in a face to make him smile but as the weeks pass, it takes more to do so. At about twelve weeks he needs to see a face which talks before he smiles at it. Speech and smiling are thus closely linked in development. Talking to each other is a social activity. It is as if he is encouraging you to talk to him by rewarding you with a smile. And he plainly enjoys it. His

smile gets broader and he wriggles with pleasure as you talk to him.

The power of a baby to engage other people in talking to him is powerfully demonstrated by the way in which he seems to encourage adults to use a special form of speech when talking to him. Sometimes called 'motherese', it is high-pitched, repetitive, full of expression and accompanied by much face-pulling. Mothers (and fathers) who use it bend over or pick the baby up so that their face is about a foot away from the baby's face. This is the distance at which small babies can focus their eyes most easily but adults seem to know this intuitively. They then launch into short bursts of 'Who's a pretty, bitty, little baby then?' and the like. It works brilliantly; babies love it. They enjoy adults directing high-pitched, rhythmic, expressive, questioning speech to them. There is absolutely no point in trying to do anything more complicated. It's what they like to hear.

You may hear 'motherese' criticised for being immature and ungrammatical. It is, of course, but it doesn't matter in the slightest. The point of it is that it is a communication, not a model of how to speak properly. At this stage communication is what counts. Providing your baby with readings of leaders from *The Times* will do nothing for his language development. Responding to his facial expressions with some affectionate silly talk in 'motherese' is actually the best thing you can do. It is not trivial.

DEVELOPMENTAL CHECKS

It used to be the case that babies were taken to a clinical medical officer in a community clinic for developmental checks at frequent intervals. In some areas this is still done by a child health doctor at a child health clinic but elsewhere the doctor will be your GP who has the advantage of knowing you and your family. The older, rather rigid, system of regular developmental checks has been replaced by a more flexible approach. Most, but not all, doctors will want to check your baby's development at eight weeks when they will offer immunisation at the same time.

IMMUNISATION

At eight weeks your baby is due for his first immunisation injections:

- 'Triple' or 'DTP' for diphtheria, tetanus and pertussis (whooping cough).
- 'Hib' against the haemophilus bacteria which is one of the causes of meningitis, pneumonia and ear infections.
- Polio vaccine.

DTP and Hib are given as injections into the baby's upper arm or thigh while polio is given as oral drops. This is the first immunisation. There will be others that are necessary which your doctor will tell you about. The next will be at twelve and sixteen weeks.

Immunisation is a wonderful thing. The diseases that it protects against can kill babies. They used to and they still do. You may have heard horror stories about the side-effects of the older immunisation agents and be apprehensive accordingly. The problem is that you may not have heard the stories about the children who get the infections which could have been prevented by immunisation. We have all become used to a world in which most babies survive and thrive. Yet part of the reason for this is immunisation which has rendered most of the childhood population immune, so that the diseases in question have become rare.

Most people in the Western world will not have seen the awful tragedy of a baby dying of diphtheria. Yet it is not so long ago that most babies who died had infections which can now be prevented. Indeed, preventive immunisation is the only treatment for diseases caused by viruses like polio since antibiotics do not work on viruses. Some people say that they feel that immunisation is not 'natural' and that their baby would be better off without it. Yet these are often the same people who make sure they themselves have their 'jabs' before going off to exotic parts of the world for their holidays and hope that a vaccine for AIDS will be discovered soon. And natural things are not necessarily safe, whether they be laburnum seeds or meningitis bacteria.

You may also not be aware of the recent advances made in vaccine preparation. Modern vaccines are very much less likely to cause side-effects than those of ten years or so ago. The risks from not having your baby immunised are greater than any miniscule risk from the immunisation. Although many mothers expect some side-effects from an immunisation, these are unusual beyond some grizzliness extending into the next day.

If you or your husband have a family history of fits or seizures it is usual practice to give your baby paracetamol (Calpol) for two days after the immunisation to keep his temperature down.

YOUR WEIGHT

Some women are lucky enough to return quickly to more or less the same size and shape after pregnancy as they were before.

However, many women put on more weight during pregnancy than is strictly necessary. At six weeks after having a baby, about half of all new mothers will have a stone to lose in order to regain their pre-pregnancy weight. It can take a long time to come off. Others put on comparatively little during their pregnancy but put it on while they are breast feeding. Either way, the temptation is to try to shed it as soon as possible. Pictures of media stars 'back in shape only three weeks after her baby' don't help. However, now is not the time even to try.

It is usually quite difficult to lose weight while you are breast feeding. You will be hungry because you need a little extra food to make the milk and you may have specific cravings, particularly for sweet things. You will also be terribly tired! Dieting as well as dealing with a new baby will just make you miserable and, if you're like most women, you probably won't manage it at this stage. Remind yourself that people who are losing weight feel less cheerful than those who are maintaining a weight. Is now the time to start feeling less happy? Feeling better about being thinner will not, at this stage, outweigh the mood change which is likely to supervene if you start losing weight now.

Put the flab problem out of your mind until your baby is six months old. Only if you are still more than about seven pounds overweight at six months should you put yourself on to a serious diet or book into Weight-watchers.

No well-bred husband would dream of commenting adversely on your weight just after you have had a baby. Remind him of this. Try to make yourself feel better about your current size by smartening yourself up. That way you are more likely to collect a few positive remarks about yourself. The alternative – dressing down to the level of a lumpen slob and acting out the way you feel – ought, in theory, to elicit reassurance and expressions of sympathy but actually doesn't work too well. More usually it is just a way of punishing your self-esteem. If you feel that needs deflating, go for it. Otherwise, put on a show at the size you are.

If you can possibly afford it, go and buy some clothes for yourself (not your baby) that are not too tight. Struggling into trousers with the zip undone and a nappy pin holding them together at the top is just as depressing as still having to wear maternity clothes when your baby is six weeks old. Be very careful that your body posture does not reflect the fact that you might feel lumpy – make sure you stand tall with your tummy muscles in and your shoulders down and back. It goes without saying that you must find time to wash your hair, have it cut and put on reasonably clean clothes (the ones without regurgitated milk on the shoulder).

Continue to be aware of your body posture, not only because this will make you look better. Maintaining a good posture is central in avoiding aches and pains. Your posture reflects the way you feel but by improving your posture you feel better. Try to walk 'tall' with tummy held in and shoulders dropped. Check your posture in shop windows when you take your baby for a walk. Inspect other pram pushers critically: have they grasped all this?

THE ELEVATOR EXERCISE

You should now have your pelvic floor under something resembling control. Once you can stop the flow of urine during a pee you can start the elevator exercise. Contract your pelvic floor muscles in stages. Start by pulling up to the first floor, hold momentarily, then to the second floor, hold and relax. When you have mastered this, add the third floor, so that you go up in three stages. But instead of relaxing completely after reaching the third floor, hold and then go down in two stages. The going down bit is rather more difficult so only pause once.

It goes without saying that you will be continuing your 50 pelvic floor flicks a day and your contractions can now be sustained for a count of ten. Keep working on your pelvic floor until it is perfect – why settle for less? (see Appendix 7). This usually takes about six months (less if you had a Caesarean).

THINKING AHEAD ABOUT RETURNING TO WORK

Some people have no choice as to whether or not to go back to work. Others have the luxury of a choice but do not know if it is the right thing to do. One of the most difficult decisions that a new mother has to make is to decide whether she is the type of woman who wants to be at home with her baby while he is growing up, or whether she is happier working. There are no rights and wrongs in all this, and it is difficult to know which group you fall into until you have had your baby. Even then, you won't necessarily know what is right for you until you have actually tried returning to work. For some women, full-time motherhood is just not for them. The guiding principle is that a happy mother is usually a good mother, and there are those who are not happy unless working, just as there are women who are only happy if they spend all their time with their baby.

There is no single right time to return to work though a good piece of general advice is between six weeks and six months. Within that range, it seems to us that the optimum time for most mothers is three to four months after birth, once their babies are sleeping through the night (or at least most of them).

If you are breast feeding and are going to hand the care of your baby over to someone else, you will need at least *three weeks* to wean your baby on to a bottle. In other words quite a lot of planning ahead is needed, and even if you still have another four weeks at home you will need to start replacing a breast feed by a formula feed. Even if you are normally level-headed and logical, be prepared to feel a little sad and guilty when you start to wean from breast to bottle. For many women, having to curtail breast feeding earlier than they would have liked to is one of the most distressing aspects of returning to work. However, at the age of six weeks breast milk has few nutritional advantages over modern formula milk and the slight difference has virtually disappeared by five months. It really isn't necessary to keep disappearing into lavatories to express your own milk into a bottle. If a return to work means that you have to move on to bottle feeding with formula milk it will neither impair your relationship with your baby nor prejudice his A-level results. You can, of course, still continue to breast feed your baby in the evening and morning.

If you want to continue breast feeding at work, have enough money and a sympathetic employer, the ideal arrangement is for a nanny to bring the baby to you. The alternative – disappearing from your desk every four hours and fighting through the traffic to arrive home tense and tight-lipped – is dismal and not worth it.

The real problem of returning lies beyond the practical arrangements. When you are preparing to go back to work you are likely to feel you are being a bad mother. You may panic that you have made the wrong decision, even if it has been made for you. In any case, you will probably be seriously worried as to how you are going to cope on very little sleep. But most of us can afford to have the odd morning when we function a bit below par and the strange thing is that usually no one notices – we set higher standards for ourselves than are set for us by others. It is a worry which, although having some basis in reality, is fuelled by wavering self-confidence – a common enough curse of new motherhood. Curiously, more sensible concerns occupy less mental space. For instance, are you sure you can fit into your work clothes? It may be necessary to go and buy some to tide you over until you have completed shrinking back to a pre-pregnant shape.

You will probably feel guilty at leaving your baby (especially if you have had to wean him because of your work) and anxious for his welfare. At any point, you may think, something dreadful will happen to pay me back for abandoning my baby. Yet you will probably not voice such concerns openly because you know in your heart of hearts that they are irrational. Awkwardly, this makes them persist and keep you in a state of vulnerability because you are unsure whether you are doing the right thing. You do need the opinions of others to provide you with some support.

The odds are that your mother did not return to work after having you as early as you have done. This means that she is not in the best position to offer the empathic reassurance and advice which would support you emotionally. It has even been known for the occasional new grandparent (whether a blood relative of yours or not) to make a critical remark about where they think your priorities should lie. Your sensitive hearing will pick up even the mildest adverse comment from others (especially relatives). The best defence is to have the unequivocal support of your husband – emotional and practical. Make contacts with other working mothers who will support you and, in turn, feel supported by you. Immerse yourself in their values and learn some practical tips from them.

Practical support from your husband comes down to the mundane. What you really need now is a wife. It may be a little tricky to sell this idea to your husband. Perhaps he'll read this page. What he is going to have to do is more than pay lip service to your return to work. He will have to listen to your agonising about your decision. And then there is the shopping. There is a whole raft of drudgeries to do with running the house, not all of them fascinating, which he will have to take some responsibility for. You need him to do this uncomplaining (just like a wife).

Consider the advantage of a bleeper or a portable telephone so that your nanny/childminder can reach you anywhere. Although expensive, the latter will do marvels for your state of mind, particularly if you are caught up in traffic on your way home.

If it's too difficult, think about whether you really should be going back to work now. You're in control and perhaps you can put things off or even give in your notice. There is no absolutely right thing to do and it may be better to fix a later date in your mind for going back. The important thing is to plan rather than drift or panic. We have given the topic of returning to work quite a lot of space because it is so challenging for those who are going to do it, but that doesn't mean that everyone has to do it. You might appropriately make an active decision not to do so or not to do so until . . .

It is, of course, possible to write an entire book (or two) about the whole subject of working mothers and the necessary childcare arrangements so we haven't gone into practical details. It may be reassuring to read one or two books now, so the transition feels less daunting. Those that we like are listed in Appendix 10.

STAGE 6

Back in the fast lane and picking up speed

17

Three months onwards

This section concentrates very much more on you as the parents (and especially you as the mother) than the baby. He will change enormously now and quickly learn an amazing number of skills – including putting everything into his mouth. All of this you will probably monitor with the help of a baby book, and you will check his progress against your friends' babies in spite of your secret conviction that he is streets ahead of every other baby.

At about fourteen weeks, you are likely to start feeling less tired and rather more in control of things. You have, in fact, survived the worst of the sleep deprivation and your quality of life should be improving. By now you may have a baby who settles at about 7 o'clock in the evening and thus have a little time for yourself. But, in spite of this, you may find it surprisingly difficult to use the time for creative leisure opportunities. A number of women may secretly be feeling seriously drained and flat. Looking after a baby is an awful lot of work and even though your baby will be the best thing that has ever happened to you, getting through the days can seem a bit of a slog. Thinking back to how things were before you were pregnant may induce a sensation of unreality – was it really once possible for you to do a full day's work, go for a swim and then out for dinner? You have become a skilled mother but you will not yet have picked up the threads of your earlier life.

Your husband is back at his work and has probably re-engaged in it as much as he was previously. He has accommodated to his baby and accepted his new status as a father. For him the baby is (a wonderful) part of the home set-up and you might be secretly irritated that for him it has all been rather easy *and* that he can get away from it all. If his work means he has to spend time away from home, you might also be alarmed to discover that you now feel uneasy in the house at night on your own.

To you he probably seems much less engrossed by your baby and less involved in babycare than you are. He may let slip that he is a bit fed up at your preoccupation with the baby and would appreciate your rediscovery of sexual recreation. But for you sex is almost certainly not at the top of your list of priorities and quite possibly not on it at all. He wants to know why you have changed, whether and when you are going to be your old self again, and he might even accuse you of being boring. Indeed, at times you may feel a little jaded or even bored yourself.

Yet there are some extraordinary moments of pride, love and satisfaction. What began with a show is now on the road and gathering speed. At some stage in the next few weeks you will realise that you have accomplished the tasks involved in the first part of becoming a parent. You will be establishing yourself as a mother as well as a wife and a woman. You aren't ever going to be your old self again; you are going to be your old self transformed.

GOING BACK TO WORK

There are good studies that demonstrate that having a working mother does no harm to a child and if she has a satisfying job which boosts her self-esteem, then her child will benefit indirectly. Children's self-esteem derives principally from their parents' self-esteem and an adequate sense of self-worth is an important element in preventing emotional complications during development. Of course, for a number of women, bringing up a baby is a rewarding task in its own right and they will derive more than enough pride in themselves from just that. But there are others who need the stimulation (or the money) gained from paid work.

Working women are less susceptible to depression, so a mother's return to work may also prevent her becoming depressed, which again is good news for the baby. All this, of course, hinges upon his childcare arrangements during the day being adequate; but then that is what most working mothers are concerned to get right.

When to return

There are two reasons for saying that it is best to get back to work before your baby is six months old. Firstly, if you leave it too long, you become immersed in babycare and lose your confidence for work-related things. Secondly, at about six months of age, babies begin to cling to their mothers and cry bitterly at separation from them. This is normal and signifies their development of a selective emotional attachment to you. It will happen, whether or not you return to work, and will apply to separations around the home (such as your going to the loo). But if you start leaving the house to go to work at the same time as your baby is beginning to show separation anxiety, you will find the wrench almost unbearable. All your guilt buttons will be pressed simultaneously.

Childcare arrangements

Decisions about childcare revolve around a number of considerations. One of these is where your baby will be while you are working. If he has a nanny, he will be in his own home. If he goes to a childminder, he will be in her house. And if you belong to the tiny minority of women who work somewhere that has a crèche, he will travel to and from work with you.

No one of these alternatives is automatically superior. Each has its own pattern of advantages and disadvantages. Nannies are convenient but expensive and usually live in with you which can cause the occasional problem in its own right. As your baby grows older, meeting other children at a childminder can be a bonus for their play and social development. Crèches are undoubtedly convenient but can also be wearing because you find yourself popping in and out during the day. A crèche is also a caring environment for a number of bacteria and viruses who will appreciate your provision of a host for their own breeding activities.

If you can afford a nanny, well and good, but many women will use a childminder during the working week. There will almost certainly be a local grapevine to be tapped when you are looking for one. Otherwise, all childminders must register with their Local Authority Social Services Department who will keep a list you can have a look at.

If you are very organised, you will find someone available to look after your baby at weekends too so that you can have a rest or find time to go out with your husband *à deux*. If you are lucky enough to have grandparents living nearby who offer to look after your baby, do use them. By definition they have brought up at least one baby, are safe, and will play an increasingly important part in your baby's life.

Remember that what you need to look after your baby is someone who is used to babies, sensible, kind and competent, no more than that. You don't need the services of a consultant paediatrician to look after a baby – even your baby. Nevertheless, plan to spend as much as you can afford on a nanny or childminder (or crèche) because you won't be able to relax unless you know he has the best you can afford. *Never* economise on childcare.

Should you be freelance and working at home, don't fall into the trap of thinking you can work and look after the baby at the same time; you won't be able to concentrate. You won't do either job well. You will still need some help with babycare if you are going to be any good at your job. It doesn't mean that you are a better person if you can just about stagger through being both an exhausted, distracted mother and an exhausted, distracted money-earner at the same time.

In fact there is a principle here: compartmentalise things and try to create some boundaries around your responsibilities and activities. You *can* do several things at once and sometimes this is the right thing to do. But you may also find this means that those several things are not done well. You do need to see your husband separately without the baby being there too; you need to provide your baby with undivided attention from time to time; you do need time on your own so that you can be all the things you are apart from a mother. If you are at work, then you need to concentrate on work.

Full-time or part-time work?

If you can, try to return to a part-time or flexi-time commitment. Curiously, most women find working three or four full days and then having a complete day off easier to manage than five short days. The reason is that each day when you leave work you are actually coming home to even more work. The impact of this transition is greater than the burden of staying at work for the extra time.

There are going to be days when you have to take time off because your baby is ill or you need to take him to the doctor for an immunisation or developmental check (if you don't do this yourself, you get a black mark from your doctor). If you are still trying to do your previous full-time job but compressing it into a part-time framework of three or four days you end up with an overpacked diary. In such circumstances, having to take a day off in an emergency is a nightmare which you can avoid by moderating your ambitions and not cramming appointments end-to-end into your diary. You may have to wean yourself off ambitious workplans to give yourself some flexibility. Be prepared for your employer to become a little grumpy if you have to take time off for a sick baby – after all they interviewed you for the job and estimated your fitness for it, not your baby's. You may feel it wise to put in a few extra hours at some stage to compensate for all this.

MAINTAINING YOUR RELATIONSHIP WITH YOUR HUSBAND

The opposite of undivided attention is divided attention. There is a sizeable chance that your husband is experiencing your divided attention for nearly all the time he is with you. Babies are experts in attracting attention and accordingly will muscle in on any act whenever they have the chance. They are often quite greedy about it too. Your baby is not likely to say, in so many words, 'Go, on, talk to him, don't mind me. I'll amuse myself quietly for an hour or so.' Yet somehow you have to deal with a husband who is likely to be feeling excluded from your attention and affections, who can feel irritated by this and may be almost as tired as you are from getting up at night. Somehow you need to manage to give your husband your undivided attention from time to time. And he needs to manage to do the same to you.

Think of yourself as a photographer with a camera which has a zoom lens. With the lens set at a wide angle you can include everyone in a shot. On close-up, one person fills the screen. If you are like most new mothers, you will spend much of your time alternating between close-ups of your baby and wide-angle shots which include your husband too. Should this be the case, remind yourself that there are two more shots you need to include.

One is the close-up of your husband. He needs at least an hour or two of your undivided attention each week. In order for this to happen, you will both have to get away from your baby to allow yourselves to go out together for a walk or a meal. Try to do something specific with this time or you might fall asleep.

The other is the close-up of yourself. You continue to need some time and space for yourself to maintain your old interests, to look after your appearance and to remind yourself that you are someone in your own right as well as being a mother. If you can do this, you will be attractive and interesting to your husband (and, indeed, to anyone) rather than the reverse – which can happen.

In order to take a close-up picture of yourself you need

to do one of two things. On a camera you would activate a self-timer which might remind you that the essence is planning time for yourself. Alternatively, someone else would hold the camera. This could be your husband. He needs to give you some undivided attention. Are you making it possible for him to do this?

He can take the baby off your hands for extended intervals and will probably relish the pride which goes with sole responsibility for that time. It is different from tagging along with you and the baby all the time which can easily make him feel spare.

If you have weaned your baby then there is an opportunity for both you and your husband to get right away. You will certainly not scar your baby for life if you both bunk off to a hotel for a night or two, leaving him with his grandparents or live-in nanny. Some people also discover that leaving their baby with their parents for a couple of nights may cure an otherwise stubborn bad sleep habit. Going off for a week's skiing is probably less of a good idea, though. If there is a person who suffers, it is going to be you – racked with guilt and separation fears. Babies are well able to tolerate separations from their parents in the first five months of their lives, though from about six months they start to develop an emotional attachment to you which means that they will become anxious and distressed if you leave them.

None of this can be reduced to a simple formula. People are different and some fathers like being part of a family while others enjoy being on their own with their babies. The important thing to bear in mind is that sometimes only one person should be in your viewfinder, rather than you unthinkingly maintaining a wide-angle perspective all the time. In the latter instance everyone experiences divided attention.

MAINTAINING YOURSELF

Getting some rest

By sharing the babycare duties between you and your husband you can each get some sleep during the day, at least at weekends. He takes the baby out while you take the phone off the hook and crash out. Later, you do the same for him. With this in mind, be cautious of going away to stay with friends or family at weekends. If you are not in your own home, it is much harder for each of you to peel off in turn from the socialising. Do not despair about your fatigue. Your energy levels will eventually come back to normal (until you get pregnant again).

Getting organised

Much of this book is about planning, managing and getting organised and you may have skipped some of it if you find all this a turn-off. But if you are going back to work at this stage, getting organised is essential. You simply have to make arrangements ahead of time instead of being reactive to circumstances. Diaries, lists and time-management techniques generally are all crucial for your survival.

Maintaining your networks

Although it is important to get out of the house from time to time, the advice not to go out socialising two nights running is so important we are repeating it. It's often very difficult to decline an invitation on this basis, especially if your self-assertion skills are not yet up to capacity, but don't get bullied into accepting. Babies always seem to sense that you have had a late night by choosing to have a very early morning. It's extraordinary how quickly even friends with children of their own can forget how necessary it is for you to make sleep a priority in these first few months. Once again, you need the unequivocal support of your husband in this.

If you are not working, make a special effort to keep up with girlfriends. Organise alternate morning child-swaps. In particular, try to make a point of seeing those who stimulate you.

If you are having people for dinner, you don't need to prepare a gourmet meal. Cook something which is easy to prepare: a leg of lamb or something cold can be just as good as tasty morsels *en croute*. Have the confidence to keep everything very simple and expend only minimal effort on preparation. Don't apologise, serve good wine and keep the baby out of the way most of the time.

MEDICAL CHECKS

When your baby is twelve weeks old and again at sixteen weeks, his second and third immunisations are due with further doses of DTP, Hib and oral polio vaccine.

You may notice that the rate of his weight gain slows down at about this time but this is not likely to be a cause for alarm if your baby is well in other respects.

WEANING ON TO SOLID FOOD

Most women start their babies on solids at about twelve to fourteen weeks. Babies need to start on solid food somewhere between three months and six months – not before. Breast or formula milk will give your baby all the nutrition he needs for up to six months; therefore it is not in your baby's interest to give him anything else before twelve weeks (or fourteen weeks if he was premature). There are some very heavy and/or hungry babies who are the exception to this, and if you think you have one of these, discuss the matter with your health visitor or GP.

One of the objects of weaning is to encourage the natural progression from sucking to chewing – it is not to 'fill him up' so he sleeps longer during the night! Solid food, therefore, is always offered from a spoon and never put into a bottle. Babies take some time to master this new technique and will sometimes bite the spoon by mistake, so you may want to buy a special plastic type without sharp edges.

It doesn't really matter what you start with – most mothers try baby cereal or jars of puréed fruit bought from the chemist. Introduce solid food slowly, a few spoonfuls before or halfway through a milk feed. Respect his taste preferences and the inevitable conservatism of babies; it is best not to introduce a new food more often than once every two days – otherwise if there is something that doesn't agree with him, you won't know what it is.

Initially, it is better to start with bought food rather than something you have lovingly prepared yourself and puréed. There are two reasons for this. Firstly, baby-food manufacturers are good at knowing what babies like, which is important if the procedure is to be a pleasurable experience for you both. They have to be careful that their food has all the appropriate vitamins in too, so don't worry on that score. In any case, at the moment your baby is just learning a new skill, rather than being dependent on solids for his nutrition. Secondly, for the first week or so, he will be taking such small quantities that you will find yourself throwing away quite a bit. No one likes throwing away food that they have spent time (and love) preparing so you may be tempted to 'encourage' your baby to take more than he wants and subsequently put him off the whole business.

Ordinarily speaking, you don't have to think about adding vitamins, iron or fluoride supplements to a baby's diet until he is six months old.

DUMMIES

Earlier in this book we advocated a dummy as a useful way of helping your baby to soothe himself so that you did not have to do this for him. From about four months on a baby can put his fingers or thumb in his mouth so that he no longer needs a dummy to suck for self-soothing. Most babies will therefore discard their dummies of their own accord between three and five months. A minority of babies will show no signs of this and if yours is in this category it will be up to you to try to wean him off the dummy (if you want to) by not giving it to him very often, and leaving him to use or develop other ways of quietening himself. Some babies are not going to accept this move and if you feel strongly about seeing it through (and when you feel tough enough to cope), you may have to brace yourself for a few days of protest by imposing cold turkey and throwing it away.

SLEEPING

It has been said that you love your children in direct proportion to the amount of sleep they allow you to have. You might empathise with this.

With a bit of luck, a fourteen-week-old baby will be going through the night without demanding a night feed though may be waking earlier than you would like. If he is still waking in the small hours, try to substitute a bottle of warm fluid other than milk for night feeds (baby fruit juice, fennel tea or bottled water). Take alternate nights on duty with your husband and sit it out. Your first duty is to survive, not to try to change your baby's night-time habits in a fruitless showdown.

In general terms, the problem begins to shift from crying at night to difficulty settling him at bedtime. The first thing to do is fix a bedtime at a point in the evening when you are likely to win. Make a decision as to when night starts and fix a time for this. A good guide is when your baby finally settles after an early evening's activities but you need to balance this with what is convenient for you and compromise accordingly. Be cautious of the dictum that the later you keep him up the easier it will be to settle him and the later he will sleep in the morning. Unfortunately, this theory yields unpredictable results in practice. Try to stop him falling asleep in the late afternoon and watch out for the common problem of a father returning from work and hyping his baby up by boisterous play.

If you can, always try to settle him in the same room but not with the same level of ambient light. Allow the room to be darker at night than during the day (not usually too difficult). That way you can set the environmental cues for him to recognise both that he is expected to go to sleep and whether it is appropriate to go back to sleep should he wake.

Because babies can't tell the time, it might be worth establishing other evening rituals which act as cues that bedtime is approaching, such as a bath, followed by putting him into a nightdress (a more specific cue than a stretch suit which may seem to him just like another of the babygros which he wears during the day) and a special lullaby. Such routines act as a reassurance to the baby because he knows what sequence to expect and they thus also act as a communication as to what he is expected to do next.

You might want to include a feed in the routine but don't let it end up with him falling asleep at the breast because he needs to develop the skill of falling asleep alone. In the middle of the night the owner of the breast will be getting her own sleep and it will not be there for him to turn to for help in falling asleep.

PARENTING

You are now a parent but not necessarily a confident expert on babies and childcare. You will receive a ton of advice, much of it delivered in certainties such as 'You must...' or 'Never...' or 'They always...' Be sceptical; most of it is pretty poor and contradictory.

Some of the findings from the systematic study of child development are a little surprising and overturn what would appear to be received wisdom or the assumptions that many people make. Before you take too much advice on board, perhaps we can draw your attention to half a dozen broad principles of parenting in the light of what is known about child and parent development.

1 *The first duty of a parent is to survive.* The most important responsibility towards your baby is to be available, not to rear the perfect child (thank goodness). This doesn't mean that you have to remain physically close to your baby all the time, rather that you should be a constant and generally available figure

throughout your child's life.

2 *Parents are perfect if they are 'good enough'.* They don't have to get everything right as luckily babies are, by and large, parent-proof. You can make mistakes and it won't matter much. In any case the influence that ordinary parents have on the development of their children is rather less than most non-professionals think. This is just as well, as most parents cannot actually be entirely in control of their own lives, let alone manage to be utterly consistent and all the other wonderful things that perfect parents are supposed to be. If parents can keep their child and his best interests in mind, be sensitive to his experience of the world and respond appropriately to his needs as a separate person (and see point 6 below), they are doing sufficiently well.

3 *It's not what you do, it's the way that you do it.* Attitudes and relationships count for more than procedures and practices. For instance, from the point of view of your baby's personality development, it doesn't matter at all in the long term whether you breast feed or bottle feed. As a rough rule of thumb, a parent who can provide love for the child as he is, coupled with a measure of respect for him as a separate person, is going to do the right thing in terms of handling the child. Exactly what she does is less important than establishing a loving relationship between her and her child.

4 *You can't judge your worth as a parent just by the development or behaviour of your baby.* Babies are individuals from day one and have a say in their own development. Some aspects of development are beyond the power of parents to influence. Gender is one, of course, but the baby's early temperament is another.

Some children are born difficult. You may be an outstanding parent but still have a child who misbehaves in a supermarket from time to time. Often you have to do what you think is right even if it doesn't have an immediately rewarding effect on your child in the way you want. Do not be afraid of your own experience, judgement and authority. In all of these respects you are ahead of your child and you should stay in charge. Stick to your guns and don't look to your child to provide reassurance that you are doing the right thing.

5 *Look after yourself and your marriage as well as your baby.* Babies and children are only passing through your life. They are only on loan to you. If you sacrifice yourself completely to their needs so that you have no time for your husband, you may lose him and therefore rob the child of his father. In a similar vein, if you are, by the time your baby is a young adult, a mother and nothing else, your offspring's departure from your side and entry into the wider world will seem to him and to you to be impossible because it will rob you of all that you are. He will feel too guilty about this to abandon you. You will not have reared an independent person. Parents who live vicariously through their children run the risk of producing children who feel they have to satisfy their parents rather than live their own lives.

6 *Do as you would be done by.* By and large, if you do what seems to you to feel right, to be reasonably safe, and do for your baby what you would have liked to have done to you when you were a baby, then you won't go wrong. Be faithful to your own intuition, it's what it is there for.

7 *Don't get hung up on having to get it all perfect right from the start.* Continuing processes count for more

than beginnings. We don't think perfect starts are that important and we have argued that no one has sufficient control over the process to achieve one in any case. We do try to tell you how to make it more likely that all three of you get off to a good-enough start – which is what really matters.

CODA

At some point round about now it will dawn upon you that you have come through. Life without your baby now seems unimaginable; it is as if he has always been there. You have admitted one more relationship into your life and you now have a real family. In the last few months you will have learned things about your baby, yourself and your husband which you never knew you didn't know, and you have become a more complex person, more mature and wiser. Colic and patchy nights permitting, you will also be a more satisfied one, too. Thus you have achieved your role transition: you have become an established mother as well as a wife (and all the other things). From now on your confidence in your new responsibilities will grow and your energies return. Enjoy your baby, enjoy yourself.

Appendices

1

Maternity nurses and nannies

Most women cope without a maternity nurse but, if you have the financial resources, employing one lightens the load considerably. This might be very important if you know that you need to return to work before nine weeks, and your job requires a particularly alert mind. If you have twins, the case for having a maternity nurse is much stronger. Bear in mind that the cost on a week-by-week basis may well be the same as your mortgage. Have you got room in your house for her?

You will need her from the time you come home for a total period of about four weeks. This is enough to give you a flying start but not so long that you become dependent on her and lose your self-confidence. It isn't usually long enough to establish your baby in a routine if you are breast feeding, in spite of claims to the contrary.

If you know of a particular nurse through friends, fine, book her well in advance. Otherwise contact a nanny agency as soon as you can (at about six months of pregnancy) as the demand for maternity nurses exceeds supply. However, should you have unpredicted twins or a very difficult baby it is sometimes possible to get a short-term maternity nurse at very short notice.

You must interview her. She will be living with you so you must get on with her. Don't employ anyone you are frightened of! Ask about her qualifications. There is no single qualification for a maternity nurse. The most highly qualified maternity nurses will be State Registered Nurses (SRN), some of whom will have a midwifery qualification (SCM) as well. They will have been trained to look after you as well as your baby whereas nursery nurses (NNEB) will have had a training which is focused mainly on babies. Check out her availability and what the arrangements would be if the baby arrives much earlier or later than the EDD.

If you are like most women, you will find the prospect of interviewing a maternity nurse quite daunting. You know that you are the employer and should be explaining what you want but, if it is your first baby, you are unlikely to be absolutely clear as to exactly what it is you do want when put on the spot. Think about having your husband or a friend with you, particularly if, like very many pregnant women, you find yourself uncharacteristically indecisive. Tell the agency your specific requirements beforehand so they can send someone sympathetic to your needs.

Sort out with the maternity nurse by discussing at the interview just what she expects to do herself and what she expects you to do in the line of general household work. What facilities does she need in order to do her job and what does she want for herself? Will she, for instance, help with all the family's ironing or just the baby's clothes? Will she shop for the family? Who will prepare her meals (is she vegetarian)? Consider carefully whether you want her to eat with you. You may well want her to take the baby away from you in the evenings so you can eat together with your husband.

Beware of those who promise that they will have your baby sleeping through the night and/or in a four-hourly breast feeding routine before they leave. For the majority of babies and mothers this is only possible at the expense of establishing an adequate milk supply for the future – the babies might well 'sleep through the night' (not be fed) or feed four-hourly, but what usually happens is that the mother finds her milk supply is insufficient for her baby within two weeks of the maternity nurse leaving.

Establish which babycare tasks she will undertake and which are down to you. Where does she expect the baby to sleep (see page 103–4). What will happen about night feeds if you are planning to breast feed – will she wind and settle your baby after a feed or does she suggest a bottle (and is that what you want)? Say what you want for yourself and your baby. Check out references by phone after the interview and ask to see another applicant if you do not see eye-to-eye with her. She may be grateful for this too.

The best maternity nurses tend to be those with a gentle and flexible approach who will adapt to your baby and to you supportively rather than trying to impose their own routines. They will, for instance, insist on taking the baby so that you can get a rest in the afternoon but will not monopolise the baby for themselves at other times. They recognise how vulnerable and indecisive even the most competent women can feel in the early weeks after giving birth and are careful not to undermine them.

If, in spite of feeling you have made the right choice at interview, you find your nurse's presence undermining rather than boosting your confidence, always remember that you are the boss and it is your baby. It is extremely unlikely that your feelings about what is right for you and your baby are going to be wrong. Talk to your husband and ask him to take the matter up with her if you don't feel that you can.

Later on, if you return to work, you will need to think about substitute childcare. Much of what we say here about maternity nurses applies to nannies. This is a large topic which extends beyond the period we are concerned with. You may like to read further (see Appendix 10):

Childcare Options in the '90s, by Penny Sparke (London, Optima).
The Good Nanny Guide, by Charlotte Breese and Hilaire Gomer (London, Century) – contains useful information about maternity nurses.
The Briefcase and the Baby, by Amanda Cuthbert and Angela Holford (London, Mandarin) – for nannies themselves as well as parents.

2

Layette (small baby gear)

- V-shaped pillow or three extra pillows for feeding
- Low nursing chair
- Dimmer switch or side light with low wattage bulb for baby's room
- Heater with thermostatic control for winter babies
- Plug-in baby alarm
- Nappies
- Supply of nappy bags
- Pack of muslin nappies (necessary for mopping up sick)
- Two plastic changing mats (one upstairs and one downstairs)
- Barrier cream for baby's bottom – zinc and castor oil or Sudocrem
- Drapolene or Metanium cream in case of nappy rash
- Portable changing bag
- Baby lotion, cotton wool balls and wipes
- Bath/large washing-up bowl or baby bathing sponge
- Infacare/baby bath solution and baby soap (Simple soap)

- Plastic-backed apron – for bath time
- Hairbrush and baby nail scissors
- Moses basket or carrycot
- Pram with cat net (small mesh will keep wasps away)
- Bouncing chair – the simplest design without a rigid back
- Car baby seat with inset to support his head
- Carrycot anchor straps and internal harness if it is to be used in the car
- Three receiving/swaddling sheets
- One shawl
- Three sheets for crib/Moses basket and pram
- Underblankets (e.g. old towels, to go *between* the mattress and the sheet).
- Three blankets for crib/Moses basket and pram – wool and/or cotton cellular
- Two soft towels for the baby's use only
- Four to six cotton vests (over the head type are easier than front ties, and some mothers like those with poppers between the baby's legs)
- Four to six nighties or babygros
- Cardigans
- Socks and bonnet
- Bibs with waterproof back

Keep all your receipts and do not unwrap clothes until needed!

3

Big baby equipment

CHANGING TROLLEY

These are units with a flat top surface for the changing mat and shelves and drawers below for clean nappies and other washing clobber. Unfortunately, most custom-built changing tables are far too low. The top should be at the same level as the mother's waist, to prevent low backache. A chest of drawers or a small table with a shelf below will do just as well – finding something the correct height is far more important than whether or not it has specific nooks and crannies for cotton wool balls.

BABY BATH

These are fairly bulky, and as you won't be using a bath for more than a few months, borrow from a friend if the offer arises. Otherwise, try to find one that hooks over the sides of your own bath as this will bring your baby up to a better height (back care again.) Some adult baths are fitted too close to the wall to allow the hooks on the baby bath to latch on safely – check this beforehand.

SLINGS

The principle of a sling is a good one but it is surprisingly difficult to find a really satisfactory one that suits both baby and mother (fathers generally need them later). Consider what it should be able to do.

It should contain the baby and steady his head in order to free your hands. You wear it on your front so that you can talk to your baby. Only when he has developed proper head control (at about five to six months) will you be able to put him in a backpack, a different thing altogether and much more suitable for fathers and walks outside.

The sling must be the right height – if too low, the weight of your baby will make your lower back arch in just the same way pregnancy does, and therefore give you low backache. The best test for height is whether you can easily kiss your baby's head. Look for adjustable shoulder straps or other ways of adjusting the height (some models have complex backs which perform the same function).

Slings are not essential. Their real value emerges if you use public transport a good deal. Some manufacturers claim that carrying your baby in a sling does wonders for your mutual relationship. There is just a little evidence to support this from one study but the effect was small and only applied to a small number of babies. Unfortunately the rather good (but extremely expensive) sling used in this study (Snugli) is no longer in production. It is certainly not worth buying an inferior sling and giving yourself a strained back in the cause of furthering your relationship with your baby if the consequence is that it is too painful to pick your baby up at other times.

BOUNCING CHAIR

Essential equipment. These are the simple chairs formed by fabric stretched over a springy metal frame. They are comfortable for the baby (whereas car seats typically are not) and prop him up so that he can see what is going on and where you are. Even very small babies can be wrapped up and put in one. Alert and energetic babies learn to bounce themselves in them so they should not be placed where they can nudge the chair off a table. The simpler the design the better. Contrary to general advice, the basic type with a simple fabric sling will not damage your baby's back. Paradoxically, the more expensive type with the reinforced or stiffened backs are much less comfortable.

DETACHABLE CAR SEAT

These are really only fit for safe and easy transport in – and in-and-out-of – cars. Used simply for this purpose they are brilliant. In the home they are too rigid for small babies to sit in for long and many babies will start to cry after about 20 minutes seated in one. Because they do not mould themselves to the baby's shape, babies will slump and their heads can adopt terrifying angles with their bodies. Small babies cannot shift their position and may find themselves glaring at the floor quite quickly. This combination of discomfort and restricted vision may be the reason why many babies in such seats learn to catnap, something which disturbs their sleep–wake routines.

MOSES BASKET

Not so much a rival to the detachable car seat as something to have in addition. In it, your baby can sleep lying flat while you move him from room to room. If you are going to take him with you when you go out to friends then there is nothing better. The problem with a traditional carrycot is that it is very heavy. When used in a car it will need both an internal harness to restrain the baby as well as external fixing straps.

PRAM

For tiny babies, a pram is better than a buggy, though buggies which have a pram-like body may be effectively the same thing. If your house can accommodate it, then the bigger pram the better because you can put shopping in it. The trays under buggies never seem to be big enough and you can't see your handbag. You won't want a pram if you have steps or stairs to your front door. Ideally the pram should fit into the hall and the sitting room and be easy for you to bounce while stationary. The handles should be at the height of your hip or waist (you will still, in theory, have a waist) and no lower.

COT

Most mothers transfer their babies to a cot at about three months. It is worth investing in as sturdy (and thus expensive) a model as possible as it will double up as an early morning playpen. Toddlers tend to abuse cots by jumping up and down and vigorously rattling the bars, so you will want to check stability and that the drop-side mechanism works impeccably. They will also use the top rail as a teething bar. For these reasons, second-hand cots are not the bargain they might seem.

BABY ALARMS

You may not need one. Most mothers can hear their own baby crying at vast distances but you may be more relaxed if you're not continually straining to listen. Be prepared to spend in order to get one that works. Expensive ones that plug into the mains electricity sockets are usually the best. Cheap ones are really very likely to go wrong or just not work.

ELECTRICAL ROOM HUMIDIFIER

This may sound unnecessary but actually they are very useful indeed if your baby tends to develop frequent colds or coughs. Humidifying the air in a room soothes inflamed airways and thus facilitates breathing. Pifco make a good one.

4

What to pack for hospital

You will need two holdalls: a small one for labour and a bigger one for your stay in hospital. The latter can be kept in the car until you are actually in your bed in the postnatal ward. Extra pillows for labour may also be invaluable, but leave them in the car too until you need them.

LABOUR BAG

- Nightdress – for early labour and/or after you have given birth. It will need to be lightweight cotton, T-shirt style with a front opening for breast feeding.
- Lightweight dressing gown and slippers (espadrilles are fine).
- Sponge bag containing washing equipment, toothbrush and paste, lipsalve, make-up (if used), hairbrush and a towel.
- Evian atomiser and elastic band to tie back long hair.
- Contact lens case and glasses.
- Watch with second hand for timing the contractions.

- Personal stereo and magazines.
- Ice-cubes in thermos flask.
- Pants – paper or J-cloth.
- Camera.
- Sweet biscuits (for after the delivery).
- Anything else suggested by the antenatal classes you attended.

OVERNIGHT CASE

- Nightdresses – two more (if staying in hospital three days).
- STs, breast pads and nappies.
- Three nursing bras and spare pants.
- Towel and baby soap.
- Baby clothes if not provided – swaddling sheets and vests or nighties.
- Fruit juice or mineral water.
- Hairdryer – for episiotomy stitches.
- Stamps, cards and address book.
- Telephone money or card.
- Knife and scissors (for fruit and flowers).
- Tissues.

PUT OUT AT HOME (FOR YOUR HUSBAND TO BRING)

- Baby car seat.
- Clothes for you to come home in (maternity size!).
- Clothes for your baby to come home in – if not already needed in hospital.
- Shawl for baby's journey home.

5

Circumcision

The foreskin (loose skin over the head of the penis) can be removed by someone who knows what they are doing. Babies have relatively large foreskins. If done for religious reasons, it may be cut off with a knife. For other reasons, a plastic clip is clamped on so that there is no blood supply to the foreskin which then drops off after a few days.

Bear in mind the following points:

- There are no medical indications for routine circumcision. Routine circumcision was popular earlier in the century because it was thought to be 'hygienic' or to prevent cancer of the penis, but the national paediatric associations in Europe and America no longer hold this view and advise against it.
- Although some circumcised fathers worry that their sons will want a circumcised penis in order to look like them, logically this would best be left until the son is old enough to decide for himself.
- As far as we can tell, it hurts just as much when you are small as later on in life (it has been studied as a severe

stress event in research on infant psychology). It may be even more distressing when you are a baby, as no one can explain to you what is happening or reassure you that the pain will stop.
- The tip of a circumcised penis is less sensitive in later life
- It is a surgical operation which can go wrong (for a few babies each year in the UK).

If you have had your son circumcised already, so be it. There are no long-term emotional complications. Otherwise, you can guess that we are against male circumcision unless there is a specific medical reason for it – and there hardly ever is in babies (a tiny number of older boys will need circumcision for recurrent infections beneath the foreskin). We similarly do not recommend female circumcision, tattooing babies, scarring their faces for cosmetic reasons, binding their feet, or leaving them exposed on the sides of mountains overnight. There have been, or are, societies in which such practices have been sanctioned because they were thought to be a good thing and parents worried whether the children would be affected if they didn't carry them out.

6

Postnatal exercises

Lie on the floor with a pillow under your head. Begin and end each exercise with a pelvic tilt.

BASIC PELVIC TILT AND PELVIC FLOOR

With knees bent, flatten your back and relax. Now flatten your back again, pull up your pelvic floor, relax your pelvic floor and relax your back.

SIT UP

With knees bent, flatten your back. Rest hands on thighs and breathe in deeply. Breathe out while lifting head and shoulders to slide hands to knees. Hold for a count of five, then lower. Repeat three times.

HIP HITCHING

Lie *with knees straight*, feet pulled up towards face. Keeping the small of your back on the floor and knees straight, shorten and lengthen alternate legs. You should feel a pull in your groin.

After three weeks ...

LEG SLIDE

With knees bent, flatten back and keep it flat. Breathe out while lifting your head and keeping heels together, slide heels away from your bottom and return them (the return journey is more difficult!). Put your hand between the small of your back and the floor to check that your back is always squashing your hand.

DIAGONAL SIT UP

With knees bent, flatten your back. On outward breath, lift your head and shoulders and take the left hand to the outside of your right knee. Repeat three times on each side.

CURL DOWN

Sit *with knees bent* and feet on the floor. Drop chin on to chest, keep your back round and straighten arms. slowly uncurl backwards as far as possible twice. *Do not* fix your feet under furniture or allow your knees to straighten.

Always hold your tummy in when standing and walking.

7

The perfect pelvic floor

All women benefit from a strong set of pelvic floor muscles. It is their future insurance against stress incontinence and prolapse (see page 31). After childbirth it is quite possible to restore the muscles to a state as good as or even better than they were before pregnancy.

Keep doing your pelvic floor exercises (50 contractions a day) until the muscles are in perfect condition. It will usually take six months to rehabilitate the pelvic floor following a normal delivery and three months following a Caesarean section. You will know you have a perfect pelvic floor when you can:

- Maintain a contraction for a count of 30 seconds.
- Take your pelvic floor up five floors and down four floors (see page 183–4).
- Stop the flow of urine midstream – however full your bladder.
- With a full bladder, jump with your legs apart, cough and remain dry.
- Make your husband squeak.

When you can do all this, continue the exercises at maintenance level as a daily 'well-woman' exercise. Muscles that are not used regularly will weaken and waste. Try to do at least ten contractions a day, combining both 'flicks' and sustained contractions. This means a daily routine of around eight quick flicks and one or two contractions, each maintained for a count of ten. Programme yourself to do these when stuck at red traffic lights or when you find yourself standing in a queue. Remember that neither your abdominal nor your buttock muscles should move at the same time as your pelvic floor.

8

Is my baby ill?

If you are on your own during the day with an unhappy, grizzly baby you will feel appallingly responsible for the decision as to whether to call in the doctor. You don't want to be labelled overprotective but you are apprehensive.

You can buy a very good kit called Babycheck (from the Child Growth Foundation – see Appendix 11) which is essentially a sophisticated score sheet of the signs of illness in a baby. It will tell you when to be appropriately concerned. Alternatively you can rely on simple rules of thumb:

- If you are gravely worried, then something is likely to be wrong (mothers are usually right in this respect).
- Sick babies go off their feeds.
- Blood from anywhere is serious.
- Breathing difficulties are serious.
- If in doubt, call your doctor.

It is normal to panic about the possibility of cot death. It is extremely unlikely to happen. The term 'cot death' covers a number of causes for babies dying unexpectedly; there is no single cause. You will have done as much as you can do to minimise the chances if you do the following:

- Put your baby down on his back with his feet near the bottom of the basket/crib (so he can't wriggle down beneath the blanket and has space to wriggle up before colliding with the top end).
- Don't wrap him up in too many clothes if the room is heated. This is particularly important if he is unwell. His head needs to be exposed so that he can lose heat.
- If his mattress is partly plastic covered, put a thick underblanket under him as a further measure to prevent overheating.
- Don't smoke.
- Call a doctor if you are worried that he is ill.

Department of Health guidance is to put a baby down on his back and recent evidence suggests that this is even better than putting him on his side, probably because some babies will roll from side to front-lying. Below three weeks this is not an issue; indeed new babies settle more readily when put on their side. The main thing is not to put him down on his front, though from about four months on he may roll on to his front spontaneously during sleep. It doesn't matter if he does; at that age you don't have to roll him back again.

If your baby is snuffling with a blocked-up nose and struggling with learning how to breathe through his mouth you will be worried. Feel free to check him frequently or keep him in your bedroom until he picks up again. In such circumstances being a little 'neurotic' is perfectly healthy.

9

Accidents and basic principles of first aid

This is not meant to be a full account of everything that can go wrong with your baby. For that you need a baby book. But there are some principles which you should consider as part of assuming parental responsibility. Firstly think about safety and avoid unnecessary accidents. With this in mind, there are two items of equipment you absolutely must have:

- A child's safety seat for the car. If you have a carrycot not only does the cot have to be strapped in but the baby has to be strapped into the cot as well. Not surprisingly, carrycots in cars are not as popular as they used to be.
- Smoke alarms for the baby's bedroom and the landing outside. This is terribly important as you cannot rely on the baby crying until it is too late.

There are several common and avoidable causes of accidents in the first six months:

- Someone drops the baby or he falls off a surface.
  - Let children know that they must not pick up the baby if there is no adult present.
  - Do not put bouncing chairs on tables or worksurfaces because vigorous bouncing causes them to move.
  - Never leave the baby unattended on a changing trolley, even if the phone goes or the doorbell rings. He can roll. Take him with you.
- The baby chokes on a small object. Babies who have learned to pick objects up transfer them to their mouths to find out about them. Keep a wary eye on what the baby can reach and prohibit other children from giving him sweets or peanuts.
- Burns from overhot bathwater, a kettle on a worktop which is pulled over, or a drink which has been heated unevenly in a microwave and has hot spots even though the few drops you test don't seem to be too hot.
- Drowning, especially if left momentarily in the bath (NEVER do that).
- Overheating in a parked car in sunlight or an overhot bedroom.

Always take a baby to hospital if he has:

- Fallen, hit his head and been knocked unconscious.
- Swallowed something dubious. If you know what it is – a plant, berries, pills or whatever – take a sample with you to the hospital.
- Been burned (while in transit, keep the affected part cold by immersing it in water and ice).
- Breathing difficulties.

10

Further reading

The Postnatal Exercise Book, Margie Polden and Barbara Whiteford (London, Frances Lincoln Ltd).
Childcare Options in the '90s, Penny Sparke (London, Optima).
Executive Mother, Jill Parkin (London, Hodder & Stoughton).
Juggling it All, Sarah Kilby (London, Vermilion).
The Briefcase and the Baby, Amanda Cuthbert and Angela Holford (London, Mandarin) – for nannies themselves as well as parents.
The Good Nanny Guide, Charlotte Breese and Hilaire Gomer (London, Century) – contains useful information about maternity nurses.
Babies, Christopher Green.

11

Useful addresses

Child Growth Foundation (for Babycheck)
2 Mayfield Avenue
London W4 1PW
Tel: 0181 994 7625

Mam (UK) Ltd (dummies)
Unit 2, Priory Road Industrial Estate
Priory Road
Aston
Birmingham B6 7LG
Tel: 0121 326 6992
They will know your nearest Mini Mam stockist.

National Childbirth Trust (for breast pumps)
Alexander House
Oldham Terrace
Acton
London W3 6NH
Tel: 0181 992 8637

Working Mothers' Association (general information)
77 Holloway Road
London N7 8JZ
Tel: 0171 700 0281

Index

abdominal muscles 24, 29, 30, 35, 92, 125, 230
   arrangement of 35–6
   exercising of 38–9, 92, 125, 135
   lifting and 39–40
   pregnancy and 36–8
accidents, first aid 233–4
afterbirth (placenta) 64, 66, 67, 80
anaemia 99
amniocentesis 57
antenatal classes 23–8, 78, 125, 166, 167
   exercises in 24, 29, 33
   hospital and 23
   purpose of 23–4
anti-depressants 171
Apgar scoring 64
attachment 72

baby alarms 53, 221
baby bath 217–18
'baby blues' 93, 97
Babycheck kit 231
back problems 34–8, 92, 110, 217, 218
   bathing and 91–2, 217
   dishwashers and 40
   nappy changing and 128, 217
   posture and 39
   sleeping and 43
bathing
   baby, positions for 130–31
   mother and 91–2
bedtimes 203
birth 63–8
   baby's appearance 63, 65–6, 81–2
   complications of 75–6
birth weight 87, 108, 115
bonding 11, 17, 64–5, 69–72
bouncing chair 174, 219
bowel opening 79–80
bottle feeding 54–6, 66, 85, 91, 109, 115–16, 126, 128, 129, 205
   routines (6 weeks on) 172
breast feeding 54–6, 66, 84–90, 93, 101, 105, 109–14, 121, 126, 128, 129, 134, 149, 151, 167, 171, 182, 205
   afterpains and 91

duration of 88–9
frequency, routines, timing 87–8, 111–12, 126, 149–50, 153–4, 172–3
latching on 84–6, 90, 112
one breast or two 87
positions for 89–90, 110–11, 126, 156–7
problems of 112–14
pumps and 113
return to work, formula feeds and supplementary bottles and 154–5, 167–8
supply and demand 109–10
techniques of 110–11, 156–7
brothers and sisters 59–60, 100

Caesarean section 26, 31, 80, 94, 97, 98, 99, 102, 125, 129, 135, 184, 229
candida (oral thrush) 114
careers 9, 12, 21–2
   see also work
carrycot 220
car seat 49, 98, 174, 219, 233
changing trolley 217
check-up, physical 161–2, 200
childcare 194–6
   see also nannies
child health clinic 123, 124, 179
childminders 193, 194, 195
circumcision 57–8, 124, 225–6
colds 127–8
colic (3-month) 149, 150–53, 165, 173, 174
colostrum 54–5, 84, 87, 91
coming home 97–117
community midwife 102–3, 108, 123
confidence, loss of 14, 47, 70–71, 169, 170, 186
constipation 79, 134
contraception 162

cots 220–21
cot death 106, 231–2
cradle cap 131
crying 11, 203
   causes of 141–2
   coping with 141–5
   evening fretting and 145–9, 150, 165–6
   forceful 149
   'screamers' 143–4
   wind and 142
   see also sleeping skills

day nursery 10
daytime sleeps 174–7
demand feeding 112
demands of baby 9, 10, 14
dependency of baby 9–11
depersonalisation 99
depression, postnatal 27, 125–6, 166, 169–72, 193
   anti-depressants and 171
   cognitive therapy and 171
   progesterone and 171
   symptoms of 169–70
developmental checks 179–80, 196
diet, mother's 101–2, 104, 121–2, 151, 152, 155
dummies 116–17, 145, 147, 149, 168, 202

ear infections 150
EDDs 21, 47, 48–9, 212
engorgement 86, 97
emotional fatigue 46
emotional life, changes in 46
epidural 26, 77
episiotomy 26, 56, 67, 78, 79
exercise
   abdominal muscles 38–9, 92, 125, 135, 162
   during pregnancy 29–43
   elevator 183–4

INDEX

pelvic floor and 29–34, 92, 124–5, 134–5, 162
postnatal 92, 124–5, 227–8
exhaustion 13, 99

fatigue 167–8, 169
feed-hunger cycles 178
feeding arrangements 54–6, 108–16, 153–5
    techniques 101
    vomiting and 126–8
    see also bottle feeding; breast feeding
finances, changes in 21–2
fingernails 108
fontanelles 81–2
forceps delivery 26, 66, 78
formula milk 55, 85

getting it right 73–6
Guthrie test 108

health visitor 123
helplessness of baby 10, 11
high blood pressure 18
holidays 21
hospital 63–8
    coming home from 97, 224
    labour and 49, 224
    packing for 223–4
    postnatal ward 77–94
husband
    back to work 121–2, 192
    depression of wife and 170–71
    nappy changing and 130
    night feeding and 167–8, 203
    paternity leave and 122
    relationship with, maintaining 138, 163–6, 206
    return from hospital and 97–9, 101–2, 104

sex and 162–3, 192
as support at home 47–8, 122, 146, 152, 165, 167–8, 182, 186, 187, 198, 199–200
time spent with 195, 196–8, 206
visitors and 82–3

illness, baby's 231–2
immunisation 180–81, 196, 200

jaundice 82, 88, 93, 101, 114

Keilland's forceps 78, 135

labour 23, 45, 63, 73, 78, 79, 91
    medical intervention and 24, 25, 26
    'natural' 24, 25, 26, 73
    pain relief 23, 25
    techniques 24, 25
layette 52–3, 215–16
lifting 39–40
lines nigra 92
lochia 68, 80, 124, 134

mastitis 155–7
maternity bras 56, 86
maternity leave 17, 21
maternity nurses 48, 93, 97, 134, 161, 211–14
meconium 82
milia (spots) 106
Moses basket 53, 220
'motherese' 179
mother/wife/parenting role 12–13, 14, 19, 45–9, 163, 192, 207

naming 56–7, 83
nannies 10, 11, 168, 185, 194, 195, 198, 211–14
nappy changing 128–30

night sleeping 175–7
nipples
    cracking in 113
    shields for 113
    soreness of 88–9, 112–14
    see also mastitis

pain relief 67–8, 79, 86, 91
parenting 191, 204–7
    attitudes and 205–6
    'good-enough' 205
    survival and 204–5
    yourself, marriage and 206
paternity leave 122
pelvic floor muscles 30–31, 78–80
    arrangement of 32–3
    exercising 30–34, 42–3, 68, 79, 99, 124–5, 134–5, 162, 183–4, 227–30
peri-anal haematoma (piles) 78, 79
personality, baby's 73–6, 136–41, 143
    difficult 137–9, 140–41, 164
    parenting and 73–6, 138–40, 205–6
    placid 136, 140, 141, 164
phenylke tonuria 108
physical tiredness 20
planning/thinking ahead 7–8, 10, 14–15
    depression and 169
    your baby and 51–8
    yourself as new mother 45–9
    your other children 59–60
PMT 20
postnatal depression *see* depression
postnatal ward 77–94
posture 39–43, 183–4
    bed and 41–3
    cars and 41, 42
    dishwashers and 40
    lifting 39–40
pram 220
pregnancy, changes in late 19–20
premature babies 19, 69–70
primary maternal preoccupation 20
prolapse 31, 34, 229
pyloric stenosis 127

recovery 79–80
relaxation tape 167
rest
    afternoon 19, 123, 162
    daily 18, 19, 167, 199
    on coming home 100–102
room humidifier 128, 221

sex 94, 124, 135, 162–3, 169, 192
sleep
    deprivation of 19, 45–6, 134, 162, 167, 191
    getting sufficient 122, 202–4
    see also bedtimes
sleeping arrangements, baby's 53–4, 103–4
    choices of 103–5
    evening fretting and 148–9
    lighting and 105, 203
    positions for 106–7
    see also temperature
sleeping skills 144–5, 174–5, 177, 204
sleep-wake cycles 176, 219
slings 218
smoke alarms 233
soya milk 115
squint 108
stimulation 133
stitches 67, 68, 78, 79, 102–3, 124, 134, 162
stress incontinence 31, 34, 229